# What others are saying

"A must-read for EVERY contemplative woman — whether pre, post, or slap-dab in the middle of LIFE!"

---Alinda C. Sledge, MSW, ACSW, LCSW
*Professor of Social Work* and
*I Can Cope Cancer Support Group Coordinator*

"A rollicking account of a woman who, in spite of being tormented by midlife frustrations, discovers her path to peace and purpose. This is a book we can all learn from!"

---Tracie Maltezo Henry
*Tri-Girl Publishers*
*Editor of the Seaside Times*

"Establishes kinship with the millions of women experiencing midlife transitions of their own by taking them on the author's journey in a humorous, courageous, and poignant way."

---Ken Berk
*Film Producer*

"In the authors evolution, she becomes real.  I marvel at her ability to amuse, share openly and encourage others."

---Kyra Gordon
*Jackson, MS*

"On first meeting Sallie, I confess I suffered from the usual male condescension toward beautiful women — all curves and winsome smiles, but don't bring up Plato or Kant if you want a straight answer. Then I read the proofs of this book and was stunned by her intelligence and understanding of the human problem. I had apologies to make and hereby make them. This book is the work of a gorgeous and intelligent person."

Bern Keating
Author and Renowned World Traveler

# Unplugged...

## at last!

Kerry + Dave,
Keep the Faith!

Hulett Sallie

# Unplugged...

at last!

The Flip Side of Midlife Madness

By Sallie Astor Burdine

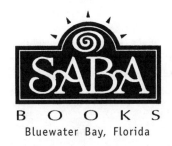

SABA

B O O K S

Bluewater Bay, Florida

Published by:
SABA Books
P.O. Box 5265
Bluewater Bay, Florida 32578

http://SABABOOKS.com

Unattributed quotations are by Sallie Astor Burdine.

Library of Congress Catalog Card Number: 2001116838
Burdine, Sallie Astor

UNPLUGGED...at last!
The Flip Side of Midlife Madness

1. Midlife
2. Inspiration
3. Women's Issues

Production by Tri-Girl Publishers
Cover design by Pearl and Associates, Inc.
Back cover photograph by Elizabeth Watson

Printed in the U.S.A.

ISBN 0-9705464-0-8

To my mother,
Jane Astor,
who taught me to rely
on the infallible truth of
"This too shall pass"
and
to the memory of my Mother-in-love,
Baby Jane Burdine,
the epitome of an unplugged woman.

# *Thanks*

*To Bern Keating, acclaimed author and dear friend...* First, you believed in me — which was all that truly mattered. Next, you showered me with your expertise and encouragement for which I will always be grateful.

*To Ferris Frost, professor of writing and author...* For not turning me away, but so generously getting me started.

*To Tracie Maltezo Henry, editor, graphic designer and Godsend...* Thank you for your expertise, your patience and your friendship.

*To the friends who hung in there* — *always inquiring about "Unplugged" year after year after year...* **Audrey Gluschke**, for her belief and confidence in me; **Judy Jernigan**, for her love and encouragement; **Julia Peabody Potter**, for her thorough work at reading and proofing; **Alinda Capps Sledge**, for her professional advice and her openhearted consistency.

*And a special thanks to Mary Ellen McNamara Hammett...* For insisting I take this book off the shelf, for helping me keep it alive, for the endless hours of reading it over and over, and for her inspiration when words eluded me.

*And as always, I want to acknowledge...***Hank,** my knight in shining armor, and the three treasures I cherish most in life... our children, **Matthew**, **Ben** and **Jane Alden**.

# Contents

Our deepest fear is not that we are inadequate.

Our deepest fear is that we are powerful beyond measure.

It is our Light, not our darkness, that frightens us.

We ask ourselves, who am I to be brilliant, gorgeous, talented and fabulous?

Actually, who are you not to be?

You are a child of God.

Your playing small doesn't serve the world.

There's nothing enlightened about shrinking so that other people won't feel insecure around you.

We were born to make manifest the Glory of God that is within us.

It's not just in some of us; it's in everyone.

And, as we let our own Light shine,

we unconsciously give other people permission to do the same.

As we are liberated from our fears,

our presence automatically liberates others.

Nelson Mandela
*1994 Inaugural Speech*

*Introduction*

# *Plugs*

I remember when Bob Dylan and Eric Clapton first came out with their new *Unplugged* releases. I bought them immediately, for I was thrilled with the possibility of hearing the simple beauty of their acoustical guitars, voices, lyrics and songs. When I listened, I was not disappointed. Without all the electrical instruments, synthesizers, mixers, and other plugged-in "extras", their music could be appreciated with a new clarity.

For many women, midlife is similar to becoming *unplugged.* The experience will vary — depending on how willing and brave we are as we go through the process. Even so, we all have the opportunity to begin anew with a certain clarity and beauty as we allow the extra, unnecessary plugs in our own lives to be removed.

I can imagine these musicians, as youngsters, playing their wooden guitars at home alone or jamming with friends. Then, as their age, success, and talent increased, so did the amount of backup instruments and singers. Even their own guitars became electrified. Speakers, microphones, extension cords — you name it — wires, plugs and sockets were everywhere.

Such were our lives as little girls. After being umbilically *unplugged*, we remained free of expectations and pressures, and most of us lived our lives as carefree children. The onset of puberty, however, begins our own experience of increasingly becoming plugged-in.

Why is it that we women seem to resemble an electrical socket from the day we cross the physical threshold from child to woman? The onset of our menses is, perhaps, a cruel, yet appropriate, analogy for what is to come. Our young bodies suddenly become receptacles for cotton corks and unfamiliar pads that act as sponges between our legs. This is merely the beginning — the physical manifestation of having to plug-up our most private parts.

Some of us were without a clue as to what to expect when we first started menstruating. Thirty to forty years ago, when we midlifers were about to "start", sex education was not even a concept. Many of our mothers were reluctant to talk about "the curse". My mom gave me a little book when I was about twelve. I was horrified. *I'm going to do what? Start bleeding all of a sudden one day, in my panties — at school or some other public place. Yikes! What if someone sees? And I will bleed for a week every month for the rest of my life?* (My book didn't mention menopause.) *And why?* (My book also didn't mention sex.)

Coinciding with our new need for physical plugs were the pressure plugs of our outer environment. As young teens, we were faced with new challenges on how to look and act. Our parents may have demanded one set of standards and our peers most likely demanded another. Society also asserted its influence, and, before we knew it, the receptacle of our lives was full. Or so we thought. Next came the awareness that boys had something they wanted to plug into us as well!

Yes, the options, varieties and sizes of plugs were endless. Our new awareness of boys, worries about our looks, whether to be preppy or hip, which club(s) to join — so many choices, so many plugs just waiting to empower and deplete us at the same time.

As young women, in our twenties, our menstrual periods lost their scariness, as they simply became expected nuisances. They remained uncomfortable and inconvenient, yet we learned to deal with them. The peer pressure became less threatening, as well, for most of us had adopted a certain, yet possibly temporary, style and set of values by then.

Nevertheless, there were new plugs and roles waiting to amp into us. Careers, marriage, motherhood, social pressures — just dangling before us as missing pieces of our puzzles. All of these and other issues began to increase in intensity as we kept adding candles to our cakes.

I imagine when Eric Clapton first took the risk to unplug, he was faced with many challenges to keep his music as impressive and successful as it had been.  To depend on his own talent without any backup aids must have been strange and uncomfortable at first.

We women have a similar challenge to face as midlife and menopause rear their potentially 'ugly' heads.  Some of us may take the risk by choosing to have what is becoming an all too common "recommended hysterectomy". Others may have no choice — as the "recommended" is a life or death "requirement", as in my case. But ultimately, menopause is a sure thing for all women and it can be strange, uncomfortable or downright terrifying.

Menopause arrives in our lives with its own irony — similar, yet opposite of the irony of beginning our menstrual periods. Shock, fear, humiliation, self doubt — questions about who we are and who we will become — haunt us at both puberty and menopause. Upon beginning menses, we begin to plug-in. But upon beginning menopause, if we are paying attention, we begin to unplug.

The cessation of bleeding allows us to unplug the cotton corks once and for all.  It can also occur with the cessation of our previous fulfilled and unfulfilled roles.  For some, it will happen slowly and naturally.  For others, like me, menopause will be instantaneous as the result of a total hysterectomy, including the removal of ovaries.

But, whether menopause has arrived or not, we will all have our share of hot flashes and mood swings. Some of us will have a harder time with vanity and our fear of aging. Others with saying good-bye to previous roles or unfulfilled dreams. The intensity will vary, but we all will have a transition to make. Whether it happens before, during or after menopause — at thirty-eight, forty-eight or fifty-something, there will be an unplugging of life as we have known it.

If you are reading this book, you or someone you love is probably going through a similar midlife stage of confusion and frustration. Or maybe just a vague sense that the inner you, as well as the outer you, is changing. I hope as you read my story that you will find comfort in the fact that you are not alone. You, too, can handle the unplugging of previous connections without losing your power, energy and self. In fact, this is your opportunity to get rid of the negative and emerge with more power, as your very being becomes less loaded and less ready to blow a fuse.

It has been several years since I became *unplugged*. The freedom of life after menopause is before me now, and it is with great anticipation and relief that I enter this new phase of my life. My unplugging process was a nightmare, but what I learned as I passed through it will forever enrich my life.

I beseech you not to let your unplugging bog you down as I did. Flow with it, seek humor in it and remember that your losses will likely be compensated with growth and enlightenment.

      If you have already become bogged down, have no fear —
there is always a backup generator to help you 'rev' up again.  This
is your soul, your spirit, your faith and ability to trust in God.  It
is crucial, though, to remember that, in order to reclaim your
power and optimism, you must slowly, yet surely, allow yourself to
let go of the extra or the unnecessary facets in your life.  Resolve those issues; release those previous roles or unfulfilled
expectations.  This is when your life and the lives around you will
become more enriched with every new day.

*One*

# *Emergency*

A dreamlike awareness of warm liquid oozing out of me and soaking my underwear, nightclothes and sheets awakened me. I groggily arose to creep to the bathroom. My heart began to beat so hard that I could actually hear it within my head. Dizziness and faintness were overtaking me, but I made it to the toilet in time to sit down while my vision, equilibrium and heartbeat returned to normal.

Blood was everywhere — down my legs, all over my nightgown. A trail of red drops on the floor marked my path from the bed. More frightening was the amount of blood and clots rushing out of me into the toilet. The hemorrhaging eased up eventually, and after rearming myself with clean pads, clothes and towels, I returned to bed. Surely, the flow would diminish by morning. If not, I would call for help.

In hindsight, I should have immediately sought medical attention. However, this monthly onslaught had become an expected nuisance. Besides, my doctor had told me months before that heavy periods were common for women "approaching" menopause. Granted, I had barely turned forty, but I assumed the "approach" could last five to ten years. Little did I know my "approach" would be like the descent of an aircraft toward a landing area. "Ladies and gentlemen, we are now beginning our final approach to the International Menopausal Airport. Please fasten your seat belts."

Yes, I thought I had plenty of time before the crash landing of "Menopause." On this particular night, I believed that within a day or two the bleeding would lessen, end — and life would be comfortable again until the next cycle.

I also rationalized that seeking help would have been troublesome and hazardous as my husband, children and I were staying in a remote cabin without a phone in the snowy mountains of Colorado. We had a car, but the blowing snow and freezing conditions outside discouraged me from waking my husband and three small children to drive down that dark icy road. I suppose only women who are accustomed to dealing with female afflictions and concerned mothers could understand my rationale that night. Of course, hindsight is 20/20. If I had known my life was in danger, the inconvenience and fear would not have been an issue.

Nevertheless, morning arrived, the snow let up and my husband freaked out. It wasn't the bloody towel between my legs or the crimson-stained sheet around me that alarmed him so much as the utter paleness of my face, gums and fingernails. When I arose and my heart began its beloved duty of beating wildly in search of blood to sustain me, we knew that I had crossed the line from "approaching" menopause to a foreign and hostile land.

Upon arrival at the medical clinic, the doctor took one look at me and pricked my finger, waited five minutes for the results, called an ambulance to take me to the hospital and started me on an IV. I was medically going into shock.

After a sonogram revealed that fibroid tumors were the culprit, a D&C was scheduled to be performed immediately. I was told later that if my hemoglobin level had dropped any lower, brain damage, followed by death, would have been likely.

I was hurriedly wheeled into the operating room, where for the first time in my extensive surgical history (as you will read later) the doctor was actually ready and waiting for me! I knew then that more than just my womb was in danger. My very life was threatened. Why else would this surgeon be scrubbed and poised at the end of the operating table? This was a far cry from the notoriously busy and perpetually late surgeons I had come to expect.

The anesthesiologist, however, refused to do his job until

five units of blood arrived and raised my count to the minimum required for general anesthesia and surgery. It was hairy for a while, at least until they shaved me. Ha! But, the beautiful HIV-free (hopefully) and selflessly donated blood finally arrived, and the operation successfully, although temporarily, stopped the bleeding.

My doctor was convinced that the fibroid tumors and heavy menstrual periods would return. He recommended a hysterectomy as soon as I was stronger. So one month later, my reproductive organs (ovaries and all) were removed. Strange how these body parts that had been my allies during my quest for offspring had suddenly become my enemies. Now I was relieved to be rid of them, traitor that I am.

Thus the surgery robbed me of my internal female organs with my utmost permission. Not only was I saving my life, but I was also ending my slavery to PMS, which was increasing in intensity and duration as my "approach" continued. My victims (husband and kids) were relieved as well.

I was also pleased that I would never again have to stroll up to the checkout counter with my grocery basket full of assorted bags of pads and tampons — just as a couple of cute guys stood in line behind me. And my husband would no longer have to spend all that time on the feminine hygiene aisle looking for the "super- maxi's" in the purple bag or the "slender-mini's" in the blue box. The shapes and sizes from which to choose were becoming more mind boggling than diapers.

This is not to say that I took my surgery lightly. I just wanted to focus on the positive aspects of it. Little did I know, the negative aspects would win—at least in the beginning.

It wasn't until the removal of these intimate parts of my body that I read the complex, yet, eye-opening book, *Women's Bodies, Women's Wisdom*, by Christiane Northrup, M.D., a must read for every contemplative woman. Through it, I discovered that the surgery robbed me emotionally as well as physically.

According to Northrup, Eastern cultures have long believed that the health of a woman's reproductive organs is affected by stored memories and emotions about their past relationships. The philosophy contends that, if our relationships with others (and ourselves) have been controlled by guilt, sex, money or blame, then it is likely that our distinctly female organs will be adversely affected.

*Yikes! I must have had some lousy relationships with the shape my organs were in.* But aren't many relationships controlled by sex, money, and guilt, at least, to some degree?

The book also pointed out that it is important to apologize to and grieve for those organs that are surgically removed. One woman even said a devotion of gratitude and farewell to her uterus as the surgeon cut it out of her. (Wouldn't you have loved seeing the looks on the faces of that surgical team??)

Soon after my surgery, when my emotional state was a bit

unstable, to say the least, I did try to apologize to my deceased organs. I remember lying in bed with my eyes closed saying in a prayer-like manner, "Please forgive me, my dear departed ovaries and fallopian tubes. I appreciate all you did for me all those years. The cramping wasn't all that bad, and I forgive you for bleeding through my white Villager shorts that day at the church picnic. And to my beloved uterus that carried my three darling, noisy, messy, precious children, I want to say to you... "*Uh-oh,*" I thought. *"I've really lost it now. And not just my ovaries. I've lost my mind!"* I then had flashbacks of the wisdom teeth, and the pituitary tumor that were also yanked from my body. Was I supposed to apologize to them, too? Maybe so, but I'm convinced some parts just need to go — especially in order to make room for new ones — like teeth. My friend, Fidelia, used to say, "There ain't one of us getting out of here alive." I assume this means un-donated body parts, too.

Nevertheless, I do believe we need to be more loving and forgiving of our bodies. After all, they're in this as much as we are. Some surgical decisions must be made without delay, as in my case, but others need to be well thought out.

My doctor was right when he warned me that "instant menopause" would follow the surgery. He was wrong, however, when he assured me that hormone replacement therapy would relieve me of unpleasant symptoms.

Two

## Is This All There Is?

The phone rings AGAIN. It is one of my closest friends. I hang up bewildered AGAIN. It seems as if most of my friends, at least those who are female and between the ages of thirty-five and fifty-five, are losing it.

One has decided to pursue a career in film. She's doing it, too, with gusto. And her marriage to a neglectful husband of eighteen years is over, too. She's starting over.

Another friend rings to ask, "Is this all there is?" She's changing careers after twenty years of climbing to the top of her profession. Now she's looking for something "more fulfilling," yet, disturbingly vague.

What's going on? So many women are going off the deep end — some risking everything. Why? Are they all going crazy at the same time?

Six years ago, I felt a little crazy myself. I had just gone through an emergency hysterectomy that catapulted me into menopause at forty. I, too, had suffered through a period of immense uneasiness about my life. My whole being — body, mind, and soul — seemed to be in question.

Upon closer scrutiny, however, I realize that not all of my friends are actually going nuts. Some have already passed through the middle years and successfully maneuvered their way through their own challenges.

Other friends, mostly younger ones, are not necessarily exhibiting signs of lunacy. Even so, I sense a change in their perceptions and an uncertainty about what's to come.

Until recently, our conversations centered on our families, our social calendars, and our travel plans. Not that we were without depth. We also took seriously our spirituality, our sexuality, politics and the environment.

Now, however, I am noticing new subjects popping up and sticking around. Things like hormones, sagging bodies, plastic surgery, and concerns about aging parents — just to name a few.

I wonder why I am surrounded with women friends who are either presently in transition or have struggled significantly in the recent past. I am convinced this is no coincidence.

We are a part of an epidemic that has been sweeping across our country like some sort of influenza virus. Strange, though, that in other parts of the world, the concept of "midlife crisis" and/or "menopause" is barely acknowledged. It could be our diet, our culture, our society or whatever, but the so-called "change of life" is certainly a more recognized phenomenon in the sophisticated and developed countries of the world.

Close to forty million women in the United States alone are now between the ages of forty and sixty years old. We are a powerful group with not only vast numbers, but also the freedom to look, achieve and grow in ways that were limited for women of previous generations. But what can be an exciting period of growth is also a scary and dangerous time for women who are unprepared.

For many, it is a period when we face the loss of our youth, so some may see time as more of an enemy than a friend. The clock ticks faster. If they dare to dream, the dream takes on a certain urgency because it must come true before it's too late. While I believe it's never too late, others may find the shrinking of the time left to them is discomforting at best and downright terrifying to many.

My ever-happy, ever-stable, good friend, Tricia, called me one day to just say hello. We have stayed in touch in spite of living a long distance from one another. But over the previous months, I had noticed a certain sadness or aloofness in her voice.

When I would inquire, "Is everything okay? You sound different, kind of blue," she would assure me that nothing was wrong.

When I went to visit her, I knew that something was indeed wrong. Her eyes said it all.

"I used to live in a picture-perfect bubble," she said, "and now I feel as if the bubble is bursting. Nothing is as I thought it was and no one is as perfect as I thought they were. I'm forty-two and it's as if I'm just waking up from a dream world."

At first, I was shocked by her words. Tricia had it all. A loving husband, healthy children and a successful career. What could she feel was missing?

She said, "I watched a young mother with a newborn baby the other day and remembered the magic of those days for me. I was right where I wanted to be, doing just what I wanted to do — my dreams had come true. What makes it all change?"

On the other hand, several of my friends are single and without children. They seem to be missing something, too. They admit to coveting my circus life of tending to the needs and wants of my little tribe all day long. Other friends, with a family like mine, would give almost anything for some solitude.

Who am I? What am I here for? What if I never get married or have children? What if I never escape the needs of my children? What will I do with the rest of my life? These are the questions many women ask themselves in the middle years.

Depression and anxiety can easily take a foothold at this vulnerable time. We can feel unwanted, unattractive and burned out — all at the same time.

In my case, I felt too needed and wanted, yet without any real direction in my life.  My children used to have a favorite toy named "Stretch."  A zillion kids could pull on every part of his body and he would stretch in every direction until there was almost nothing left of him.  Just skinny straws of dough about to pop.  My nerves have felt like this on many days.  First, pliable — then volatile.  "Stretch" did pop one day.  I almost did, too.  But I'm still here.  A little stretched out, but still here.

I used to think that a "crisis" was a catastrophe.  But through my own experiences and those of others, I have discovered that a crisis can also be a stimulus for change.  Thus, a 'midlife crisis' can be a turning point that yields new potential and redefined values in our lives.

If we take advantage of this time, by slowing down and quietly listening to our lives, we may hear truths about who we are and why we are — and thus, begin to live more authentically.

The middle years tend to illuminate our unresolved issues and fears as our previous roles are often in transition at this time.  For instance, when all three of my children went off to school all day, I discovered that much of my purpose and identity was tied into caring for them.  Most of my services were no longer needed and my future role was in question.  I was glad to have some time to myself again, but I also became haunted with the old familiar questions that gnawed away at me before marriage, children and the Junior Auxiliary.

*What is my reason for existence? What are my gifts and talents? How can I make a difference?*

The questions for a single woman are not that different. She might have devoted her life to her career, whether by choice or by fate. Finding the right mate didn't happen on schedule. Her biological clock is running down, and the prospect of motherhood dwindles. Did she miss something crucial to her well being? Should she adopt a baby? Will that be the missing piece to her puzzle? These may be her questions and the answers will vary.

The point is this is the perfect time to ask these questions. Yet, our task is not to wallow in the sadness of saying good-bye to previous roles and unfulfilled dreams. We still have time to pursue that career dream, develop new talents, and even adopt that baby — if we so choose.

More importantly, the additional mileage we've traveled in life now offers us wisdom, timing and insight into what really makes us tick.

*Three*

# *Vanity — The First Issue*

*I am a woman who needs to be seen. I need it in a basic way, as in to breathe, to eat. Or not to be seen, that is the other increasingly attractive option, to give up the lifelong preoccupation of finding myself in others' eyes, the need to be taken in so that my existence is noted.*

— Nancy Friday
*The Power of Beauty, 1996*

I don't remember exactly when my looks became a source of measurement for my self- worth. I'm sure it happened gradually, as it does with most young girls, as our society so subtly and not so subtly teaches us its gauge of beauty. But, the point is, it happened. And when it did, I received my first heaping dose of what experts would now call co-dependency. My sense of well being and how I perceived the way others viewed me became copartners in crime.

My well-meaning family-of-origin even jumped in to convey the message of vanity to me, but not maliciously, of course. We mothers are not trying to hurt our children when we praise their looks more than their dispositions or when we mention their clothes, cleanliness, pimples or weight without counteracting our complaint with some sort of praise. It has been said that seven compliments are needed to counteract the destructiveness of one criticism a child receives.

Actually, my sweet mother encouraged vanity in order to help me, not hurt me. I was the most insecure extrovert you could ever meet. When I was barely thirteen years old, Mom enrolled me in the once prestigious Charm Modeling School. I didn't get very far professionally, mind you, but I did enjoy learn-ing how to put on makeup and strutting pretty clothes down runways in department stores.

My ego was starving, and the more it ate, the more it wanted. Sadly, my appetite for approval and attention would not be satiated for many, many years. I didn't blame anyone else for the emptiness within me. My parents gave me all they had to give. It was not their fault I needed more.

How could my father know that his frequent remarks at the dinner table about my eating too much were nibbling away at my self-image? He would say, "Sallie, if you're not careful, you're going to end up as fat as Aunt Gracie or Aunt Ethel."

Looking back, this puzzles me, as I was always too tall, too thin and scraggly as an adolescent. My mother even put me on a program to GAIN weight. When I came home from school, I would consume a milk shake with raw eggs and a special powder designed for weight gain. Someone told my mom that homemade Fudge would help, too, so that also became a daily indulgence. Talk about mixed messages!

And, of course, children can be the cruelest enemies to each other's self-esteem. I had a little mole (or "beauty mark," my mom would call it) on the middle of my cheek. My friends would tease me about that ugly bump on my face. At nineteen years old, I had it removed and now sport a scar to show for it — instead of a beauty mark just like Cindy Crawford's.

In later years, psychotherapy, with its usual method of "blame," revealed to me why fear of criticism and need for approval were my strong characteristics. Basically, I learned that somewhere, somehow, someone had made me think that my self-worth was tied into my outward appearance.

High School in the sixties, continued, as it probably does today, to reinforce this notion. The cheerleaders, beauty contests, etc. made us gangly girls with flat chests and braces feel inadequate and unpopular.

Puberty became my friend as it added curves in the right places. All of a sudden, boys were noticing me and the popular girls seemed to like me more. A certain, instant gratification came upon me as heads turned when I walked into a room.

After two years of college, I decided to drop out and take on the airlines. I needed glamour and feedback. At twenty years of age, I became a stewardess ("flight attendant" was not a job description then), and "Coffee, Tea or Me" was still considered the appropriate lingo for my profession. Weight and age restrictions were still in place, even though it wasn't long before laws against discrimination replaced our glamorous image with the reality that we were nothing more than glorified waitresses. Even so, back then, my job depended on my weight, my makeup and that ever-present smile that would keep passengers flying the sexy... I mean, *friendly* skies.

I went from Daddy to Delta, and the same message — that pretty opens doors — was repeated to me. My clay-like personality was being consistently molded into a package designed to please.

The strongest onslaught of reinforcement to my distorted view arrived two years later. The attack came in the form of a blind date. Ronald was cute, fun and rich. Within months, I quit my job with the airlines and for some reason we decided to get married.

Ron was a great guy, but he, like me, had been deceived about what really counts in this world where society teaches us all the wrong lessons. And when you're both self-centered, as is often the case with twenty-something year olds, it's even harder to see that the physical things in life are the quickest to fade and the least fulfilling.

Ronald's parents were killed in a plane crash when he was just twelve years old. Because of their life insurance and investments, Ronald became financially independent on his twenty-first birthday.

We embarked on a life of traveling and partying.  We entertained our working friends, who spent just about all of their vacations with us.  We had an airplane, a yacht, and a large home, complete with swimming pool, on the waterway in Fort Lauderdale.  It was a perfect resort setting.  And the guests came and came and came.

Ron told me he didn't believe in spending money on the little things, like a maid to help me change the sheets, wash the towels, clean the six bathrooms and cook for all our company.  And, of course, the guests were on "vacation," so they were ready to eat, drink and be merry.  The perpetual party with me as hostess, cook, and maid was fun for a while.  That is, until the exhaustion set in.

Another thing Ron didn't believe in was a fat, or even voluptuous woman, except, of course, where breasts were concerned.  He badgered me about staying thin.  It started on our honeymoon.  We were sitting in a quaint little restaurant in the south of France.  I will never forget the look on his face or the tone in his voice.  "Just look at us," he said with disgust, "We really need to go on a diet as soon as possible."  At least, he included himself in his declaration. The problem was that neither one of us was overweight. We were probably just beginning to look healthy as we indulged in the rich cuisine of Europe. Nevertheless, "eat less and dress sexier" became his motto for me. Maybe his ego was as hungry as mine.

Ron planned trips for us to take between visits from our out-of-town guests. To some, this lifestyle may sound exciting, but it wasn't. It was empty and I was a zombie.

About this time, the good diet doctor (or should I say "quack") entered into my life and rescued me. Ha! Amphetamines to go. I was raring to go and able to maintain my almost anorexic body. I was always in the mood to clean the toilets, then go out and party all night. The perfect hostess.

*Four*

## The Catalyst
## and the Connection

*If it is woman's function to give, she must be replenished too.*

—Anne Morrow Lindbergh
*Gift From the Sea*

In my world of illusion as the skinny, sexy, perfect wife and hostess, I was unaware of how close I was to disaster.  A nervous breakdown, followed by a stay at the Betty Ford Center or at least a twelve-step program, was certainly on the horizon. Thankfully, destiny intervened — with a love story that saved my life.

**...hot'Lanta**

Ron and I had decided to go back to Atlanta for the annual

Chattahoochee River Raft Race Weekend. We had both lived in Atlanta years before and had always participated in this event, which was basically a weekend of endless partying. I believe it has now been discontinued due to deaths resulting from drunken participants.

Ron and I agreed to help host a party the night before the race. It was at this party that a certain introduction would occur with life-changing consequences. It has been twenty years, but I can remember five minutes of that evening as if it were yesterday... There are dozens of young people dancing, drinking, laughing and talking, I can hear the music and remember the song. *I Heard it through the Grapevine* — upbeat and in keeping with the energy of the party. I feel someone grab hold of my arm and turn to see my friend Beebe.

"Sallie," she says, "come over here, I want you to meet my friend from Mississippi."

I begin walking with her toward the bar. I'm wearing tight, hip-hugger blue jeans with a skimpy top, completely open down the front except for two or three tie-dyed strings tied into bows (an outfit I wouldn't be caught dead in now unless I could do it anonymously with that same body). And then I see him — sitting at the bar, smiling at my friend. As we come closer, he looks at me. Beebe is introducing us, and I am looking into the most incredible green eyes. I'm still not sure whether it was his eyes or the combination of them with his salt & pepper hair and matching beard that held me captive for a few moments. Or was it the depth in those eyes? I felt this extraordinary connection to him. Not an attraction necessarily, but a connection. Yes, I thought he was beautiful, older and sexier than anyone I had ever met. He seemed strong, masculine and kind and I remember sensing somehow that he had a zest for life probably equal to mine.

I recovered quickly, and as usual, the "hostess with the mostest" offered to fix the eyes—I mean the *man*, a drink. Then we both went back to socializing separately. I don't think I saw him again that evening, and believe it or not, I don't remember him even crossing my mind.

He did cross my path though, about twelve hours later. He answered the door at a brunch Ronald and I attended the following morning.

"Oh, it's you," I said with surprise and awkwardness. "I met you last night. What was your name? Frank? Hank?" And before he could answer, I blurted, "This is my husband, Ron. Did you guys meet last night?"

I then introduced them while internally sensing that connection again and enjoying those eyes. *How could his eyes seem wise, kind and wild all at the same time?*

I then left them standing there and went in search of a Bloody Mary.

The brunch proceeded festively as the guests began to

recover from their overindulgence the night before. Ron and I mingled separately, as usual. And the man, who now had a name, Hank, seemed to be standing in the same lines as me for the buffet and bar. He finally suggested that I stay in the bar line and order both of our drinks while he tackled the buffet line and fix both of our plates. Little did I know or even suspect that this would be the beginning of our coupling, of our becoming *one*.

You see, I did take my marriage to Ron seriously, at least until it was all but over. Nevertheless, in hindsight, this fending for one another, as Hank and I did that morning, was the beginning of an "us" which would happen, years later, way on down a bumpy road.

We all eventually sat at the same table, eating, drinking and becoming fast friends. Ron and Hank traded funny stories, and I enjoyed meeting the other Mississippi guests. Hank invited Ron and me to the Mississippi Delta, where he was a road building contractor and a gentleman farmer. He was planning a "Pickin' Party" to celebrate the harvesting of the cotton crop. We accepted and arrived two weeks later in a place unlike any other in the world.

### ....The Mississippi Delta

Flat, endless fields of cotton and soybeans. Sunsets that could be savored until that last moment when the huge, neon-orange sun would dissolve millimeter by millimeter into the ground. And the endless parties, usually outside with a giant barn or cotton gin in the background. Mint Juleps and John Johnson's famous buttermilk drinks. Tables and tables of red-checked tablecloths filled with fried chicken and stuffed eggs. Oh, and the day lilies! Baskets of them everywhere.

The music never stopped. Son Thomas and Sam Chatman playing the Blues...the *real rotgut* Blues. And Jimmy Phillips singing *Leland's Smokin'* and *Greenville's Burnin' Down.* Muriel, a beautiful black lady playing gospel music and old favorites like *Darkness on the Delta* on the piano. It would be a while before Marc Cohn would discover Muriel and feature her in his song, *Walking in Memphis.*

Ron and I felt like we were in a foreign land, right within our own country. The people were so gracious, yet wild and crazy, too. We had a wonderful weekend. Hank had a date with *two* Southern belles (at the same time) and we all virtually burned the candle at both ends for three days. Upon departing, Ron and I felt as if we were saying a temporary good-bye to new yet permanent and very special friends.

### ....The Florida Keys

We reciprocated by inviting them all to our part of the world for a weekend in the tropics. Hank and two couples arrived in the evening. Hank's date had arrived earlier, and I remember sitting with her in my kitchen, encouraging her to become romantically interested in Hank. He had become a dear friend to both Ron and me, and my initial "connection" to him had somehow diminished. Familiarity and fondness replaced my feelings of awe for him.

After everyone had arrived, we jumped on our Striker sport fishing yacht and headed for the Florida Keys. It was a scandalous voyage, complete with drinking, laughing and shocking tour boats by shedding our swimsuits as they passed. Eventually, though, the Piña Coladas kept us naked most of the day and as I imagine happens at most nudist colonies, we became desensitized and unaffected by our nudity. Funny, when Hank and I look back to those days, we become a bit shocked by our immodesty.

Like innocent children (except for the alcohol), we skinny-dipped from dawn till dusk. It was on one snorkeling adventure, though, that Hank and I made our first connection of real depth. No, we didn't almost drown. We made a spiritual connection. Yes, naked, and a little drunk— we bonded spiritually. It happened when we simultaneously came up for air after diving down to view a statue underwater. The statue was of Jesus holding his arms up with a sign on his chest that read, "Come unto Me."

Hank and I both plopped into the Zodiac dingy and somberly looked at each other for a few moments. He finally said, "That's pretty strong, isn't it?"

I knew immediately what he meant. We both felt re-minded and a bit reprimanded by the symbol of the traditional religion in which we had both been raised.

But as we talked, we realized that the statue of Jesus also represented something more positive than mere judgment. It was our anchor, our foundation — something a lot more stable to hold onto than the fleetingly exciting yet empty and lonely lives we were presently living. We both had put God on a shelf, as so many young people do, while we experienced the carnal world. Now, at the same time for both of us, it was as if the shelf was tiring from bearing the heaviness of God. Or was it the heaviness of our hearts?

*Five*

# Someone to Watch Over Me

Ron and I went on a couple of more trips (thankfully, to cooler climates where clothes were needed) with Hank and his various dates and friends.

It soon became the norm that Hank and I would be the last to drop at night. To this day, we tend to be the last to leave a party due to our energy levels and how we both thrive on being with people.

But, back then, when I was married and Hank was just our good friend, he and I began to talk longer and later into the night — after the others had passed out — about what we really wanted out of life. Of course, this is how many an affair gets started and I suppose we weren't totally ignorant of this. We were just more aware of our need to vent.

When Ron and I took our next trip, a six-month boat

voyage up the East Coast all the way to Canada and back by way of the Mississippi River, Hank visited us in Montreal for a few days.

Ironically, this visit occurred just before Ron and I began our southern descent down the ever-winding and ever-widening mighty Mississippi. Little did I know this river journey would eventually reflect my marriage, even to the point of diluting it into life's vast ocean.

After painting the town red one evening, we returned to the marina, and everyone, including Hank this time, went to sleep. I was left alone at about two o'clock in the morning and decided to take our three dogs, who traveled everywhere with us, for a walk. It was not unusual for me to walk the dogs in the middle of the night in dark boatyards or marinas and Ron was generally unaware, at least until the next morning, of whether or not I returned safely to the boat.

On this particular walk, Hank suddenly appeared in the shadows. He began lecturing me about the dangers of a woman walking alone in the middle of the night. He expressed surprise and a little disgust that Ron would allow this. I remember being aware of this precious, unfamiliar sense of protection — of being cared for.

After returning to the boat, we sat up until dawn, talking again about what we wanted out of life. He listened to my frustrations about wanting children and a more settled life. I remember savoring this new best friend who understood and listened. But I also remember the aversion (or was it fear?) that I felt when we finally said good night and he kissed me lightly on the lips just before he descended below to his cabin.

How strange that the man who could make me feel so safe frightened me to my core with that first kiss. The timing was all wrong, of course. Maybe Hank felt a physical attraction as a result of our emotional closeness, but I did not. What I did feel was that for probably the first time in my life I had truly found what we now call a soul mate.

Hank left the next day. He hugged me good-bye and told me he would always be there if I needed him.

### ....Till the not-so bitter end

Ron and I moved on to our next port, where we had other friends waiting to cruise with us for a few days of R & R. But rest and relaxation were hard to come by for the perpetual hostess when people boarded a large boat in a vacation mode. By this time, I was spending a lot of time down below in my cabin with the dogs and my Bible, trying to get God off that shelf.

I also used this time to write my new soul-mate a letter that I felt I owed him. I explained that regardless of the closeness the two of us had experienced, my marriage to Ron would remain intact. I was committed and that was all there was to it.

Four months later, we arrived back in Fort Lauderdale.  I immediately called my parents in Miami to tell them we were finally home.

"Yes, Mom, we're finally on dry ground.  The dogs are thrilled and so am I."

As my mother started to ask about the trip and how long I would be home, Ron walked into the room and signaled me to get off the phone — indicating we were now on a budget that apparently excluded long-distance calling.  Can you imagine?  He had just spent easily over a dollar a mile in diesel to leisurely travel some 5,000 miles and now he was saving pennies on a phone bill.

Within about a week of our arrival home, our Mississippi friends (not Hank, though) called to invite us to another Delta party weekend.  I was sitting on the sofa next to Ron adamantly shaking my head "*no*" as Ron said "*yes*" into the phone.

After he hung up the phone, I explained to him, "There is no way we can pick up and go anywhere so soon after our six-month journey."

I also remember thinking that it would be potentially dangerous for me to see Hank again.

When Ron said, "Too bad, we're going," I realized we were close to the end of our relationship.

I told him, "I can't go on any longer. I need normalcy or at least, less partying, traveling and entertaining. Our relationship is in danger, my emotional and physical health is in jeopardy."

I pleaded with him not to go back to Mississippi.  We went.

## *Crossing the line*

A friend picked us up at the Memphis airport and drove us to his house in Hollywood, Mississippi, our usual stopover on our way to Greenville.  I remember feeling a little apprehensive, yet a little excited as well.  On our previous visits, Hank drove up to spend the night with us and would then drive us the rest of the way the next day.  But when we arrived in Hollywood, it seemed as if no one was sure if Hank was coming to get us.  I hadn't heard from him since I wrote him the letter on the boat, so I assumed he was keeping his distance.

Later that evening, I went out to walk my dogs before retiring and saw headlights approaching the house.  It was Hank.  My heart was bursting.  He got out of his car and saw me in the dark, just standing there, watching him.  We slowly walked to- ward each other, mumbling simple words of greeting, and then we were in each other's arms.

I don't know how long we held each other or who let go first, but I do know it was the hug of a lifetime.  One I will never forget.  One I can still feel twenty years later.  He enveloped me in an all-encompassing circle of love, protection, and warmth.  I remember succumbing and reciprocating.  We finally let go, saying nothing and went inside.

Ron and the rest of the group welcomed Hank and proceeded to party. It was as if nothing had changed yet Hank and I knew that nothing was the same or ever would be.

After the group called it a night, Hank and I went out on the back porch to admire the stars, as we usually did. The difference this time was that there were no words, no deep conversations, just us looking up at the sky and then at each other. Within seconds, our mouths met, and we must have kissed for what seems like hours to me now.

Words eventually came as the reality of the situation broke our spell. I told Hank that Ron and I were seriously talking about separating after this trip. It was so simple. I wanted to settle down, and Ron wanted to take another trip. I was tired; Ron was still raring to go. We had nothing left in common except a mutual sense of discontentment, mixed in with more than a little despair on my part.

Hank and I decided that we had much in common, but we would wait. From Mississippi, Ron went on to Texas for Thanksgiving to be with more friends and I went home to Miami to be with my family. As Ron and I parted ways in the Memphis airport, we both knew that a separation was around the corner, and I think we both felt a certain sense of relief.

*Six*

# What Happened To Happily Ever After?

I am sure that many of our friends assumed that Hank was the reason for the divorce, but he and I know differently. Yes, Hank was probably the catalyst, but the termination of my marriage to Ron was inevitable. We both had too many unsettled issues in our lives, too much growing up to do.

It would be nice to say that everyone immediately lived happily ever after, but they didn't. At least not for a long time. And in retrospect, it's a good thing because none of the participants were ready to live happily ever after.

Ron had a few more wives and divorces to go through. Hank had some guilt (about being the catalyst) to resolve within himself, not to mention a healthy fear of commitment.

And what about me? I went through the divorce stoically.

I even took less money than my lawyer advised in order to insure a lasting friendship with Ron, which by the way is still distantly intact.

Ron did give me enough money to buy a little townhouse in Miami. I moved my dogs, my stuff and myself and then proceeded to slowly yet surely fall apart. There I was, barely alive — the three "D's" — divorce, depression and drug dependency — killing me softly. How did this happen? Was it my vanity, my starving ego, my self-made ruler that measured self-worth by looks? Or maybe it was society's fault? Who knows? But, I imagine the same village that can raise up a child can just as easily tear one down.

I was eventually victorious over the three D's. It was a long, three years though. I started out with a blind psychiatrist who put me on antidepressants and offered little counseling. Even her seeing-eye dog would growl at me when I'd start venting.

I ended up with Billy Graham's son-in-law, a prominent psychologist who saved my life. He insisted that I make a commitment to see him regularly for several months, which allowed the process of my recovery to proceed with consistency.

During these months, Hank and I would often rendezvous in various places between Mississippi and Florida, but there were spells where we went our separate ways. Thankfully though, we always found our way back to one another.

## *Still crazy, after all these years*

Three years after my divorce, Hank and I took a leap of faith and eloped to Memphis. The first year was tough. In spite of my recent therapy, a certain insecurity and lack of identity continued to eat away at me ever so constantly, ever so hungrily.

All of a sudden, that beautiful, foreign destination called the Mississippi Delta was no longer a fun place to visit. It was permanent. I was suddenly submerged in Hank's world — coldly (from my perspective) surrounded by his friends, his family, his traditions, his church and his ex-girlfriends — and everyone's endless stories.

To make matters worse, I found out just months after we were married that I had a pituitary tumor that would require brain surgery and months of recovery. Hank used to joke that usually a man has to fix his new wife's teeth, but with me he had to go through brain surgery.

Our next challenge was infertility. We got through those tough years by keeping our sense of humor. I once dropped a glass test tube of Hanks' sperm sample in an elevator on an elderly ladies foot. The tube proceeded to break, and her husband bent down to wipe the sperm off his wife's shoe with the linen handkerchief from his coat pocket. I apologized and took what was left of the test tube. He stuffed his 'soiled' handkerchief in his pant's pocket and said, "No problem, I just hope it wasn't anything important."

On a lonelier mission for Hank's sperm collection, he was placed in the clinic's broom closet due to a lack of vacant examination rooms. He was doing okay until a maid with a bucket full of mops walked in on him and said, "Ohhh, I see you've got your hands full."

Sometimes, Hank would be in the middle of a road job supervising his crews. His radio (cell phones weren't in yet) would cackle and then he would hear me say, "Four to One, Four to One" (my number was four, his was one, being the boss man and all).

Soon, I'd hear Hank respond, "Uh, One to Four, One to Four, whatcha need, Sallie?"

Of course, I knew what he was *really* saying, *Don't you know I'm busy. Why are you bothering me now?* But since his entire company could hear what was being said, he'd try to sound nice.

I would then hit the talk button and say, "Get home quick! It's up!" — Referring to my temperature and possible ovulation.

At first, he'd say, "What's up?" But he stopped asking, when once I said, "It better be you that's up."

One of his workers told me later, "You must be a pretty good cook, Miss Sallie, the way Mr. Hank jumps in his truck so fast when you call!"

But the truth be known, sometimes poor Hank never got a

chance to take off his boots, much less eat any lunch.

In any event, the extra intimacy may have helped abate our problems as well, for we were always doing it — just in case my thermometer was wrong.

Another big help was the premarital counseling we received just hours before we said our vows. I remember when Hank's ex- priest from Greenville, Reynolds Cheney, who was then the priest in a big Memphis Episcopalian church, met me for the first time, which happened to be just a few days before the date we had set to be married. He was concerned, about many things, but mostly about the lack of time he had to prepare this future bride and groom whom he was about to marry.

Of course, I knew Reverend Cheney was a bit apprehensive anyway. He had known Hank for many years and probably never expected him to marry a gal like me. First, I was a divorcee. Second, I was a Presbyterian and third, I was a half-breed Yankee.

I imagine he put a lot of thought into what he could say to us twenty-four hours before we said "I do" to each other. Little did he know, what he did say would stay with us for twenty-plus years and be passed on to future generations.

Reynolds Cheney said, "There will be many days you do not 'feel' love for one another, but if you 'will' yourselves to love one another, the real stuff will follow." He was right, and to this day, Hank and I remember his advice on those few occasions when *love* may not be the truly operative word.  Thank you, Reverend Cheney.

And, perhaps most comforting of all, suddenly and graciously, the endless stories of Hank and his friends and the Delta began to include me as one of the living, breathing characters involved.  I suppose what I really needed was validation which was not an easy thing to come by — especially in a world so steeped in tradition and legacy that it often reeked of exclusiveness and aloofness.

My background, even with the status of being a third generation native of Miami, could not have been more different.  Why, my birthplace was not just a melting pot for Haitians, Cubans and Snowbirds, but (are you ready?) a harmonious haven for displaced Yankees and Rebels, as well.

Miraculously, twelve years later, with three precious children and our marriage incredibly intact and better than ever, we took a break from the Mississippi Delta.  We up and moved to a beautiful little town in rural Colorado.  Hank was frustrated with work, we were tired of crime, noise and traffic and so we split.  "No por que?" Would be our response.  Why not?

*Seven*

# New Lands

> *One doesn't discover new lands without consenting
> to lose sight of the shore for a very long time.*
>
> —Andre Gide

It has been almost a decade now since we left Mississippi,
yet I still cannot shake the Delta's influence, its penetration into
my very heart and soul. The natives would say my roots are too
shallow and are of no account. Only my husband and perhaps my
beloved late mother-in-law know that, although my roots didn't go
deep, they went wide and were fertile enough to absorb much in
the years I lived there.

Of all the contrasts and contradictions I have spoken of in
this book, the Delta presented the most to me. Through its

people, culture and weather, I felt enchanted and betrayed it seemed every day I was there.

In fact, my memories of the dozen or so years I lived there are strangely dominated by extremes. In the summer, the wasp-size mosquitoes were merciless as they sucked blood out of everyone, indoors and out. I remember trying to sleep with a high-pitched buzzing sound in my ears and then the quick sting of the bite and the slap of my hand. If I was lucky, I smashed the bug filled with my blood. If I missed, the buzzing continued.

After my babies went to sleep, I would drench them with Avon's Skin-so-Soft, apparently appalling to insects as well as humans. Sometimes, when I would hear their tormented sleep, I would sneak into their rooms, turn on the lights quickly and wait to catch the little vampires as they tried to feast on my children.

The heat, the utter stillness of air, as if one could not take a breath, was one of the worst extremes to endure. The agony of the animals still haunts me. Even in the shade, the temperature could easily reach over a hundred degrees. The horses were tormented endlessly by horseflies that ate them alive, and the dogs met the same fate but with fleas and heart worms as their terrorists.

Mary Ellen, used to say, "Well, the breeze may never blow, but at least, the bourbon always flows." That was the good news — the endless parties that probably kept us all sane in one-way and borderline alcoholics in another.

Yet, despite the burning heat and starving insects, there was a certain beauty that I can remember vividly. The flowers, especially the magnolias, could intoxicate one more than bourbon if inhaled deeply and closely.

My dear friend, Mary Ellen, and I, when we were truly being petty, attributed the narrow-mindedness of some (I said *some*) Deltans to their merely being drunk with the lush, heavy scent of magnolias.

"So drunk," Mary Ellen would say, "they could never muster up enough energy or guts to break out of their intoxicated spells." On our bad days, she and I would conspire to escape as often as possible in order to breathe other scents. Getting away, we surmised, would prevent us from being stuck ourselves in their lethargic world of tunnel vision.

### *...A friend of my own*

Of course, Mary Ellen and I were a bit biased in that we were "imports"— some would call us "new blood" — brought into the Delta by two of the most previously sought-after bachelors. She arrived on the scene about a year after me and we took to each other like magnets. I'll never forget our first encounter.

Mary Ellen and her fiancé, Warren, were cruising down the same dusty country road as Hank and me, except in opposite directions. After passing each other, our men, who were mere acquaintances, slowed their pickup trucks down and backed up 'til we were window to window. They then proceeded to introduce their new "stock," I mean *women* — similar to the way they would stop to show off the dead deer in the back of their trucks during hunting season.

Mary Ellen and I were made-up to the hilt and I imagine hair-sprayed as well, as we eyed one another while pretending not to be coughing up dust. Oh yes, two city girls like us didn't mind a little ol' dust and dirt. After all, we were Delta women now and proud of it.

At the time, Mary Ellen was twenty, I was twenty-eight. I remember being stunned by her beauty, radiance and contrasting features of dark, black hair and light, green eyes. Later, I would discover she was of Black Irish descent and possessed each and every one of their strong, boisterous characteristics.

Mary Ellen remembers being relieved that I didn't fit the stereotype of the Southern belle, and sensed we might have something in common. Little did we know how *much.*

A few months later, after she and Warren had married, we met again at a New Year's Eve party given by Hank and me. I greeted her with my usual barrage of questions all at once, "How's married life? How do you like living in the Delta? Who are your friends? What do you 'do'?" (The not yet trendy phrase "whaz up?" would have cut to the chase.)

Anyway, Mary Ellen just looked at me and once she truly

had my attention, she began to cry. Not with sobs, but with simple, quiet tears that began to mix with her mascara and run all over her cheeks.

"Okay," I said, "Let's go somewhere and talk"—which we've been doing ever since.

But that night, we talked of our mutual battle with insecurity. Being an outsider was tough enough, but being Warren's wife or Hank's wife — where there once was none — was even trickier. Our husbands had sowed their oats in our new town and there were reminders everywhere, even at that very party were many girls who had known them a bit intimately.

As silly as it seems now, Mary Ellen and I had a tough time dealing with the hugs of greeting and the "real" or "imagined" eye contact between our husbands and their many old flings.

We were also not instantly embraced in warmth by the other women who may have been insecure themselves, as they caught their own husbands eyeing the new stock in town. I, after all, was a blonde divorcée from Miami, *already!* Practically a Yankee. And Mary Ellen, well Mary Ellen was just gorgeous and not at all shy.

In fact, she has always reminded me of the song "How do you solve a problem like Maria?" from the movie, *The Sound of Music*. I can just see her parents and the Catholic nuns at her school shaking their heads at her when she walked by.

Today, almost twenty years later, Mary Ellen remains a

celebration of contradictions. I am sure she will forever be flamboyant and gorgeous, yet I am also sure that her unpredictability, (which many call *instability*), will never change, much like the Delta itself.

## ....*Predicting the unpredictable*

In the summer, there is a special magic and mystery that revolves around the Delta crops. The moods of the farmers change with the elements of the weather. In fact, the dispositions of the women, children, and communities in general are affected.

If there is a drought, then the thirstiness of the crops result in an unquenched thirst and frustration among the people. If there is too much rain, which either drowns the crops or prevents their harvest, then we watch our farmer friends as well drown in lost hopes for bumper crops. To some, this loss means no food on their tables, while to others it means unpaid bills at fancy clothing stores and canceled ski trips in the winter.

The winters of the Delta are probably as cold as the summers were hot. The only consistency is the incredible humidity. Mercifully, though, the mosquitoes become history when winter hits the Delta, seemingly instantly after a few short weeks of fall. Then come the never-ending gray skies and rain. "Gloom and doom" weather, I would call it.

One of our friends, Jimmy Phillips, is an incredible songwriter and musician. One of his songs, *Panther Burn,* about a famous Delta plantation, sums up the winters: "Black earth framed by gray sky, wild ducks flying in the frozen air."

When we lived there, my husband was a road builder whose success also depended on the elements. If it rained, which it did almost all winter, he would have to pay his crews even though there was no way they could pave or even prepare to pave in the rain. This resulted in quite a grouchy husband on a majority of days.

In defense of the Delta, Hodding Carter, Jr., winner of the Pulitzer Prize for his works on race issues, said it best in *Delta Ice: the storm of 1994....*

> *"If the Delta is overly hot or dusty or wet or barren for a time each year, it is also green and cool and fecund and bright, and who would want perfection without the intervening contrast that makes perfection recognizable?"*

It's not much different, contrast-wise, in this paradise of a valley in Colorado where we live. The weather can be as "moody as a debutante," to quote our friend, Bard Selden, from Hollywood, Mississippi. The ranchers' well being depends largely on the hay crop and cattle production. However, many of the new residents here, like us, depend mainly on our computers and fax machines to do our work.

Here, Hank and I live in our Utopia, supported financially

by the strange yet beautiful Mississippi Delta.  But guilt does creep in.  How dare we escape the mosquitoes, heat, humidity, floods and ice storms while letting the fruitfulness of its land support us?

I do know it took a lot of guts for us to leave the Delta, and we must live more simply and economically as a result.  Many accuse Hank of abandoning his roots, but he continues to return to the Delta in order to water them frequently.  Our children and our friends (even the Yankees!) are enriched when Hank's thirst is quenched, for he brings the legacy back with him when he returns.

In any event, life in Colorado was practically perfect until my hysterectomy.  Looking back, however, I was beginning to sense a certain discontentment before the actual surgery, as you will see in the following chapters.  I believe this uneasiness can hit us anytime before, during and after menopause — but we all will have a transition to make — sooner or later.

*Eight*

## Cosmetic Surgery

As you know by now, vanity had been a thorn in my side for most of my life, even before my catastrophe of instant meno-pause. This futility continued even after Hank had shown me repeatedly through the years that beauty, by society's standards, was not an issue with him. He has always liked women with "meat on their bones" and with "something to hold onto." His prefer-ence has always been healthy, natural, earthy women who wear little makeup and no perfume. Yet he picked me to be his wife — Miss Vanity herself, with a bottled-blonde head of hair and acrylic nails. So much baggage to bring into a marriage — includ-ing a personal scale that measured my self-worth by looks.

Thus, "looks" took priority over "health" in my life before becoming *unplugged*. I was more concerned that a lazy metabo-

lism would harm my appearance instead of my overall health.
Those "ideal" weight charts with a separate category for women
over twenty-five years of age always baffled me. It wasn't long
after my twenty-fifth birthday that I understood. My body
WAS changing. It's just a good thing I didn't know then about
that category for women over forty.

The prospect of turning forty never really threatened me
though, for I had already planned to counteract this milestone
birthday with a special little gift to myself. As my birthday drew
closer, Hank began questioning me on ways to celebrate.

"How about a big party or a trip somewhere?"

He knew, though, that my fortieth birthday gift had
already been decided upon years before. I had even put money
aside and had urged Hank to do the same. On previous birthdays
and anniversaries, I would tell him, "Don't buy me anything now.
Just remember what you're going to give me for my fortieth."

When the big day arrived, we told the kids we were going
on a romantic getaway and hired a baby-sitter for two days.
Hank drove me to Memphis and waited with me in the doctor's
waiting room with a frown on his face. He had long since stopped
expressing his disapproval of what I was about to do. I had told
him years before that this was the plan and that was all there
was to it. God bless him — I entered into our marriage with so
many insecurities — and he has continued to love me, not necessarily painlessly, but unconditionally. I remember him telling me

how beautiful I was when I was pregnant and weighed close to two hundred pounds. Either his eyesight was worse than I thought or he was a lot smarter than I gave him credit for.

I'm still not sure why I wanted to go through with my birthday present. I told myself it was just for me — to look rested and, perhaps, a bit younger. But you know as well as I do that I had my eyes done for one reason: to preserve my appearance. Besides, the doctor said it wouldn't hurt too badly and I would be able to go out in public within a few days. No big deal, right? Wrong.

They wheeled me into the outpatient operating room on a gurney. I asked the doctor *again* if he was sure I shouldn't be put to sleep.

"No," he said *again*, "you need to be awake so you can blink your eyes when I tell you to."

He added, "This will prevent me from removing too much skin, which could result in you not being able to totally close your eyes again."

I should have jumped off that stretcher right there and then, but the shot of Valium and Demerol were taking effect and I couldn't move, much less jump.

Unfortunately for me, moving was about the only thing the drugs kept me from doing. They had absolutely no effect on my ability to feel, and then to scream and cry. The next four hours were the most excruciating hours of my life. I am no stranger to pain, but nothing can compare to what I went through at the hand of that "highly-recommended" plastic surgeon. I later found out that he most certainly could have put me to sleep and kept my eyelids functioning normally. I thought I had researched this guy pretty well. Wrong, again. Remember this, gals, one or two recommendations are never enough when someone is going to use a knife on you.

After the surgery was finally over, Hank retrieved his sobbing wife and checked us into our room at the clinic's hotel. My eyes looked like swollen beets with black threads weaving in and out. Little did I know things were only going to get worse.

When I arrived home the next day, my children started crying at the sight of me — sunglasses and all. I told them I caught some awful eye infection while off on our getaway. To make matters worse, I could not see a thing for days, just blurry images. Reading, watching television, even sleeping became impossible. Never has healing been so slow or painful.

I don't relate this pathetic story in hopes of getting sympathy. Actually, I'm quite ashamed of myself. The pain served me right, and it probably prevented me from having a total overhaul when the real midlife madness hit.

Ironically, I had hopes of not having to wear makeup once my eyes were prophylactically secured from ever getting creases or bags. Now I must put on eye shadow every day to hide the permanent white scars on my eyelids caused by the surgery.

It is also not my agenda in telling this story to discourage women from having plastic surgery. Morally, to me, it is no different than extending or darkening our eyelashes with layers of mascara, except, of course, for the cost and potential risk.

Several of my friends have had breast augmentation, and others who seem to condemn surgical enhancement continue to buy their Wonder bras. They are all basically after the same effect — to feel better about themselves. Some simply want to look better in their clothes, others want and need ego feedback by luring the gazes of men, some want freedom to go braless without saggy breasts and those who take the surgical route do it with hopes of increasing their own sexual pleasure as well as that of their partners.

In *The Power of Beauty*, Nancy Friday sums up the situation well:

> *"Synthetic estrogen, testosterone, amazing beauty creams, revolutionary bodybuilding machinery, cosmetic surgery, none is going to disappear. In fact, they will flourish and multiply. There is already less of the moralistic condemnation of "looking good," even if it involves surgery, and there will be even less tomorrow. Healthy good looks' time has come, and they are not so much about eternal youth as about extended life."*

The point I wish to make regarding my own surgery is the lesson learned. For the umpteenth time, I learned that there is, indeed, wisdom in accepting the things that cannot be changed. And if we choose to force change, or prevent it, as I did with plastic surgery — it often involves a trade-off.  For me, where once were creases are now scars.

*Nine*

# The Fitness Center

Why is it we women (and human beings in general) are so susceptible to making trade-offs?  The classic one is "instant results" vs. "delayed gratification," like the cabbage soup diet that takes ten pounds off in ten days.  We get quick results yet we practically starve for ten days and then, within the next ten days, it all comes back.  This, instead of a long-term change in eating habits and exercise that results in permanent weight loss and good health.

I can say, though, that at least once in my life, I actually experienced the immense satisfaction that comes with "delayed gratification."  For many months just before my official *unplugging*, I made a commitment to join a small fitness center and amazingly stayed active in it for quite awhile. Ironically, the key to my success was a very plugged-in and programmed treadmill routine I did for forty-five minutes, four times a week.

I was slender and svelte and reasonably happy with my body and weight. Unfortunately, though, while physical exercise may have been the source, vanity was my motivation.

When the fitness center, which housed the magic tread-mills, threatened to close down, I took my grandfather's inherit-ance and bought it. No, not just a treadmill, but the whole fit-ness center.

First of all, I was afraid a treadmill at home would become a clothes hanger and secondly, I hoped that this new venture might solve another lifelong void in my life — purpose and meaning.

Within a week or two of becoming the official owner, a "natural, herbal" salesman came through the door with an aston-ishing new weight loss product. "Ma Huang," combined with other stimulants and appetite decreasing herbs, became my top-selling vitamin supplement. I couldn't keep it in stock. Most of my members became addicted, at least psychologically, to this prod-uct and I was one of them.

Yep, back in the saddle again. It had been ten years since my last diet pill, but the thought of more energy, less appetite and increased metabolism, in a natural, healthy pill was too hard to resist. We (me, my staff and members) all lost weight, but unfortunately, a lot of us also lost our motivation to keep exercis-ing. Popping herbs was a lot easier and quicker than the miles of hills and valleys we were averaging on the treadmills. So the easy way out won again, at least for the short term.

It wasn't long before the dangers of Ma Huang were being talked about in the news. Ma Huang is a derivative of the ephedra plant, which provides our pharmaceutical companies with ephedrine, a decongestant. It acts as a stimulant to the nervous system and revs up the heart, blood pressure, nerves and everything else.

College kids began taking it in order to party or study all night. Women like me were consuming it daily to stay slim and energetic.

Reports of heart attacks soon hit the media and those without addictive personalities were able to cease taking the wonder drug.

It was about this time that Hank and I began talking seriously about moving to Colorado and as my memberships were at an all time low, we thought it best to close down the not-so-magic-after-all fitness center.

I continued taking Ma Huang supplements for about a year. The last capsule I took was on the day before I almost bled to death in Crested Butte, Colorado. The emergency and surgeries that followed ended my second affair with stimulants. I am thankful, at least for that result.

The bed rest required for recovery soothed my obsession with false energy and worries about my weight. I was too caught up in hot flashes and hormonal adjustments to care about any-thing else.  It was a time to be lazy, to watch videos and escape into *lust in the dust* novels. Yuck.

*Ten*

# Emotional Breakdown and Hormone Replacement Therapy

Within two months after my hysterectomy, my double-edged sword of vanity returned with a vengeance. I began to fear that what I thought to be swelling was actually a permanent addition to my ex-reasonably flat stomach.

At one of my follow-up appointments, I questioned the doctor who had performed my hysterectomy about my inflated abdomen. He told me it was just scar tissue and not to worry.

"Not to worry?" I questioned. "Isn't scar tissue basically irreversible? And what about this certain thickness that is enveloping my body like a foam mattress pad?"

He looked at me with the same look of pity he'd probably given dozens of other postmenopausal women.

"You are in your forties now," he said and then added,

"This is to be expected at this time in your life."

*My God, three months earlier I was svelte and slender,* I thought.

As tears filled my eyes, I mumbled, "And why do I cry all the time?"

He looked at me blankly, as if he had never been asked this question in thirty years of ob-gyn practice.

"Just keep taking your estrogen," he finally said.

Again, I reminded him that my mother has breast cancer and wouldn't estrogen put me at greater risk?

Again, he would answer with, "Well, your chances of dying of a broken hip or heart disease are greater than your obtaining and then dying of breast cancer." *Sure hope he's right,* I thought.

I then asked him if there were any other forms of estrogen I could take besides Premarin. I explained that it bothered me to take a pharmaceutical that was derived from pregnant mare urine. With each pill I took, I would visualize thousands of horses being bred non-stop, confined to small, sterile stalls and hooked up to catheters all day. I read that the mares are separated immediately at birth from their foals, only to be artificially inseminated again as soon as possible. And the fate of the innocent, motherless foals? Well, we won't go there, for now.

The doctor, who by this time seemed a little agitated, informed me that Premarin was the only estrogen (at that time) tested enough to insure protection against osteoporosis and heart disease.

"Just don't think about where it comes from," he advised.

Strange how warm, informative and compassionate this doctor had been before he removed my reproductive organs. Now there was a certain chilliness and aloofness about him.

*Of course!* I thought, *My value as a patient went out the window — along with my fallopian tubes!*

He handed me my chart with "emotional breakdown" circled on the form.

The proceeding days, weeks and months passed slowly for me. It was as if my normal zestful self, along with my previously optimistic disposition, had been surgically removed as well.

I was utterly exhausted and began to fear my overall health and fitness was on the downhill slope — the green, bunny slope — slow and easy but nevertheless heading down. My decline seemed inevitable and possibly never-ending.

Looking back, my cold and indifferent doctor was probably right. I WAS having an "emotional breakdown." Who wouldn't? My black and white world was becoming increasingly gray. My looks, my beliefs, my purpose, and even my libido were all either fading away or contradicting themselves. I was in between being who I was in the first half of my life and who I would be for the next and final half.

I now wish the fear had not ruined the anticipation of the

new me. It affected not only me but my loved ones as well. I became a moody mom, a lazy wife, and a wimpy friend.

Scariest of all, was the return of a very unwelcome visitor from my past — depression. This almost-forgotten yet still familiar threat presented itself in the form of a bottomless well — similar to a dark abyss with very slippery slopes. This made life even more uncomfortable as I feared one slip, one stumble, or worse, one surrender could throw me over the edge.

As my foothold around the dark hole became more and more dubious, I eventually reconsidered my doctor's recommendation to take hormones. Adding to this was my ever-increasing body thickness — even my toes and earlobes were getting fatter.

But, I had one more question for him. What about mixing a little testosterone in with this wonderful estrogen? I had heard on a morning news show that many women like me, whose hysterectomies included removal of their ovaries, were finding relief in taking testosterone with their estrogen.

Apparently, without our ovaries we cease to secrete testosterone, except for a small amount by our adrenals and fat tissue. Upon further study, I found that testosterone fuels our sex drive and encourages muscle growth. Yes! Increased libido and more muscle to burn body fat. What a great solution to the mattress pad blues and postmenopausal blahs.

When I called my doctor to suggest we consider the mixture of a little testosterone with my horse pee (I mean, *estrogen*), he refused to prescribe it for me on the basis that it was more harmful than helpful.

I then sought second and third opinions and found two physicians who would recommend the combination for me. They felt that such a low dose of testosterone (1.25 mg) would not be harmful. Apparently, this is still controversial, but it worked wonders for me. It is important, though, to consult a physician before deciding if this type of hormone replacement therapy is right for you.

Through more research, it became evident that there are many choices of estrogen replacement. Estrogen derived from pregnant mare urine, which is prescribed and taken by millions of women, is not only causing unethical treatment and torture of thousands of horses, but it is unnecessary.

There are dozens of different forms of estrogen on the market, and there are other alternatives to hormone replacement therapy through certain foods, vitamins and exercise.

I strongly recommend that, if you are menopausal, you take the time to research for yourself the many risks and benefits of hormone replacement therapy. Once I found the right hormonal supplement for me, my sense of well being improved considerably. Little did I know, though, that many years later, I would develop breast cancer. So be very careful.

Dr. Susan Love says it best in her book, *Dr. Susan Love's Breast Book:*

*"I do have a problem with the idea that we're supposed to keep taking these hormones indefinitely — there must be some reason that menopause exists in the first place, and maybe our bodies really need to stop having these hormones at some point. Certainly the pharmaceutical companies have done a wonderful marketing job. Women now expect to crumble and dry up the minute they turn fifty. Menopause has been redefined as a disease of "estrogen deficiency," rather than a normal passage of life."*

*Eleven*

# Getting Real with Sex

Midlife may be a normal passage of life, but "normal" doesn't necessarily mean smooth.  In fact, I would venture to say that midlife is the ultimate roller coaster for many of us.

Everything from our hormones to our weight to our moods fluctuates, accelerates, decelerates, or just plain negates during this time — with our libidos being one of the first to go.  Especially for those of us in long-term relationships, our sex drive can simply pull over to the curb for a long rest, or worse, drive off a cliff forever.  Unfortunately, long-term can be synonymous with *stale* and this puts our midlife relationships in jeopardy of trade-off fever.

Another "trade-off" many married women (and men as well) make is infidelity.  For those cursed with neglectful mates, the temptation to succumb to instant gratification with a new lover is strong.  It takes patience, courage and a different kind of desire to communicate with our spouse about our unmet needs — especially our sexual  needs.

For instance, would you feel comfortable blurting out to your mate?

*"Honey, you don't turn me on anymore."*
Then to soften the blow you ask:

*"Could we start making-out again and possibly, begin sex with our clothes on?"*

And then, if you're really feeling brave:

*"Or how about doing it in the middle of the day... maybe even on the washing machine?"*

If he's still standing, then add:

*"And oh, honey, maybe with time, I could become uninhibited enough to show you how to really please me and you could let me learn how to really please you."*

Gulp! You may think, "not me" saying stuff like that to my husband.  But if the nerve hits you one day, be prepared.  I imagine the majority of spouses would be thrilled by the prospect of a little honesty in what is supposed to be the most intimate part of a relationship.

I finally got up the nerve to confront Hank about my decreasing libido and asked him to take on some of the responsibility for it.

There is a joke that goes something like this:

**Question:** What makes a woman frigid?

**Answer:** Marriage.

Unfortunately, this is true in most cases to some degree. Most men have a truly physical need for sex, so their desire is always there...even when their wife barely participates out of a sense of duty (or mere exhaustion, or lack of foreplay). Most men are also left-brain dominant, which means they can block out everything going on around them except for where they are focused.

The classic example is the man reading a newspaper while the wife and kids are trying to get his attention. Finally, the wife says, " And by the way, dear, the house is on fire." He mutters something like, "That's nice, dear." This is supposedly why men can achieve an orgasm in a splash and a flash while we women, who tend to be right-brain dominant, often become victims of Attention Deficit Disorder just when we most need to be focused.

The experts say that the brain is the greatest sex organ. So there we are, with our greatest sex organ thinking about a zillion things, like the ceiling needs painting or the carpet needs cleaning — depending, of course, on where one is looking.

Sometimes, we women really do try to stay focused as we moan, "Oh yes, darling!" But our mind betrays us with distracting thoughts like, *I wonder if the kids are asleep?* But we manage to control our mental sex organ again and whisper, "Yes! Yes! Don't stop!"

For there are truly times we don't want it to stop. And then, the thoughts come again. *Did I turn on the dishwasher?* Now where did that come from, for Pete's sake?

Anyway, you get the point. Hank *was* thrilled with my washing machine suggestion even though I was a bit distracted with mentally sorting colors and all. But best of all, we have started kissing again, and I mean KISSING, and what a difference this has made in our overall sex life.

Hank even said the other day, "Amazing, after all these years, it just keeps getting better." This is not to say that I have become a love goddess or a nymphomaniac. In fact, "quickies" are still a big part of our life. I suppose the quality and quantity of our sexual experiences will always be subject to change. But our sense of humor and honesty has certainly enriched our intimacy, which cannot help but spill over into the rest of our lives.

*Twelve*

## *Contrasting Images*

The first time I entered into the "trance," I was driving alone through a mountain pass in Colorado.  The road was familiar as I made this same forty-five minute trip almost weekly to the nearest city for supplies.  What was not familiar was the strange feeling that began to encompass me.  It was as if some spell had overtaken me.  My Jeep seemed to drive itself as it wound its way through canyons of incredible beauty.

Patches of snow were so perfectly interspersed among varying rock formations that one would think the snow had been placed there strategically.  Interrupting the canyons at regular intervals were forests of blue spruce, fir and ponderosa pine, with the snow again resting majestically on the dark velvet branches.

Such was my life during the lush yet rocky journey of

menopause. At times, the patches of icy conflict and the snowy peaks of revelation seemed to be strategically placed within my life — at just the right time.

I didn't feel crazy — just bewildered. And a bit frightened of the stranger I sensed living within me. Could this new "me" threaten the life I so deeply love? What if this philosophical phase was just a prelude to complete insanity? Even partial madness could be hazardous.

After all, many of my friends were showing signs of mild lunacy, depending on one's perspective, of course. Maybe they were just shifting their priorities, which is not necessarily dangerous. To the contrary, reevaluating our values is healthy, isn't it?

But, oh dear, wasn't it just last year when my cousin's seemingly "normal" wife suddenly bolted one day? She packed up her suitcase and barely said good-bye to her husband, her kids and her home. No one is still sure why she did it. Maybe it was another man or maybe it was something as trivial as dirty socks.

I don't know, but I can relate to the dirty socks. I actually considered running away myself — just for a few minutes, mind you — one evening when I awoke from another kind of trance — one of nothingness. I suddenly became conscious and realized I had been sitting on the couch for what seemed like hours, turning socks rightside out and trying to find their mates. I tell you, I went crazy.

I suddenly erupted and began sobbing and screaming at my puzzled husband and kids, "Look what has become of my life! Mere SOCKS are hypnotizing me! I can't do this anymore. I quit!"

The children and Hank just looked at each other and rolled their eyes. I could hear them all thinking, *"Here she goes again. Poor Mama."*

But to return to the moment I just described of driving through the contrasting landscape, I sensed the fear letting go of me. Then the utter peace, the assurance that yes, I am changing, but all will be well. I knew then that inner change does not always demand outer change. You see, I wanted nothing to change — my love and passion for my husband, my devotion to my children, where and how we live — nothing, except, of course, the damn socks.

So with the intruder of fear out of the way, I allowed myself to fully experience my majestic trance as if it were a gift instead of an assault. It was as if the car was floating on air instead of asphalt. Barbara Streisand sang to me from the radio:

*Just like the seasons, there are reasons for the paths we take.*
*There are no mistakes, just lessons to be learned.*
*No matter how many times you stumble and fall, the greatest*
*lesson is loving yourself through it all.*

BARBARA STREISAND
*Higher Ground* Album, Columbia

I lit up a smoke from a pack I had purchased weeks before in another strange moment. I rarely ever bought cigarettes, at least back then. I barely smoked except socially, when I would grub one from a real smoker. So, there I was, smoking in the middle of the day alone.

The music blaring, yet soothing. The windows down, allowing the cold mountain air to fuse with the hot, dirty smoke of my cigarette. Again, the contrasts and the blendings. An echo of my life since the hysterectomy and loss of ovaries had catapulted me into the forceful currents of menopause. Cold-hot, fresh-stale, happy-sad, frigid-sensual, scared-safe.

The next time my state of mind was invaded with the trance-like alien, I was in the middle of a whirlpool bath in my bathroom at home. I had returned earlier that day from an exhilarating day of snow skiing.

Always an intermediate at any sport I undertook, I defied the usual that very day by skiing black diamond slopes with moguls and all. I didn't do it with great ease and form, but I did it — and with gusto. A sense of challenge and determination arose within me as two friends, Audrey and Wendy, coached me down the steep, bumpy slopes. Another example of the power we women have to communicate and encourage one another.

But, oh, my forty-ish body felt it at the end of the day. Thus, the whirlpool. My husband out of town, the children occupied downstairs, the door locked, the cold white wine and the cigarette...again. As the hot water swirled around my nude body, my mind quieted and my senses awoke. The soothing sound of the swishing water hushed the noise of my thoughts as I again succumbed to the spell of the moment.

The contrasts returned. The cold wine cooled my throat after each drag of the hot cigarette. I looked down at my nakedness and, surprisingly, I thought how beautiful I was. I don't remember it being a prideful or vain feeling, just an unexpected image of myself. Maybe I had been afraid to look at my postmenopausal body.

A memory surfaced: I was a young teenager on the beach in Miami where I grew up. My friends and I were lying on the sand watching the boys catch the waves with their surfboards. Actually, we were "baking" on the sand, as back then "skin cancer" wasn't the spectre it is today. Smothered in Baby Oil, our bikini clad bodies shone and glistened as the sun cooked us like pieces of toast. We laid on our backs as our elbows supported our upper bodies so we could watch the surfers. One of my friends said, "Sallie, look at the muscles in your stomach!" I looked down and saw the rippling definition of muscle lying upon my midriff. Strange how little significance that sighting of my lean and slender body had on me back then.

But now, twenty to thirty years later, as I lay on my back in the whirlpool, I could not see any rippling muscles on my stomach. In fact, I could not see any muscles at all. Just soft skin and flab floating in the water. A little scar on my navel reminded me of the laparoscopy I had when going through infertility treatments. And the Cesarean scar would forever mark the birth of my daughter. Ironically, the doctor had called it a "bikini cut."

Nevertheless, I lay there admiring (or was I merely accepting?) my forty-two year old body. The awareness was beginning to dawn on me that all that I am, inside and out, is fine. So what if I can't see any muscles in my stomach anymore — I have three children instead. And even if I didn't have them to justify my jiggling stomach — I was beginning to see glimpses of accepting my imperfect body. Emotionally speaking, that meant a lot.

If I could get over attaining self-worth from the ridiculous feedback that physical attractiveness can yield, then just maybe I could conquer my self-centered need for approval and admiration in mental pursuits as well. How exciting to think that degrees, talents and masks may no longer be needed. What a relief! What a great moment that was.

And then the contrasting images began to whirl with the water. Everything was different, yet still the same. All was sane, yet insane. My body was softer, yet my mind was stronger. My soul was sleeping, yet vividly dreaming. And then the kids began pounding on the door.

My awareness of contrasts visited me often during my midlife passage. There was no real power in it, just a certain sense of well being and a resolve that contradictions are acceptable.  In fact, they are the stuff that life is made of.  Without contrast, how would we recognize the extremes or the mediocrity of our days and moments?

Knowing sadness enables us to appreciate joy. Experiencing confusion gives value to clarity.  Losing our zest for life primes us to exult when we find it again.  And what a gift it is to find sensuality after frigidity.

So, emotionally speaking, it was in the midst of my *unplugging* that I discovered what was disguised as a terrorist was really my ally.  The sadness, confusion, apathy and frigidity were just the preliminary emotions that would soon transpose into their contrasting opposites.

Music and writing probably saved me during this time.  I began regurgitating on paper everything I was absorbing with the din of country, rhythm and blues, or soft rock in the background.  Either the lyrics of the songs blew me away or the instrumentals would soothe what needed calming or stimulate what needed reviving within me.

The irony was that these two media, music and writing, also contrasted their value to me during my *unplugging* process.  They became my friends as well as my enemies in that they would also encourage a certain rebelliousness in me.  Thoughts of leaving and finding my true self teased me and tempted me.  Looking back, however, I can honestly say that I never doubted the necessity of my inner journey.  The pain didn't surprise me, but the pleasure did.  After I stopped fighting the "emerging me," I began to enjoy the process.  It was scary, but delightful.  Apprehension was soon replaced with anticipation.

*Thirteen*

# *The Great Escape*

In the midst of my *unplugging*, two of my Mississippi friends were instrumental in bringing me out of the darkness. They were dealing with their own bouts of blues, so we were quite a trio as we escaped on what was to be my first "all girl" get-away.

Mary Ellen called me excitedly one afternoon. The day before she had called in tears, frightened and worried about her father's recent heart attack. The day before that, she had called in what was becoming her usual voice of despondency regarding her failing marriage.

On this day, Mary Ellen's voice was different. I could hear hope, excitement and anticipation. It wasn't long before the tone of my voice joined in with hers. Her precious father was doing much better, but his weakened condition provided *us* with just the cure we needed.  Mary Ellen's parents' intended trip became our escape!  *Non-refundable hotel suite in New York City for three days and two nights?*  "Oh, dear."  *Top-notch theatre tickets to Phantom of the Opera?*  "Oh, my."

"Yes," I said, "Of course we can do it and so can Sherry!"

### ...."Sherry" detour

Sherry became another best friend to me in the Delta, even though she belonged to Hank first.  He was actually in love with only her photograph, which sat on his mama's counter for three months before they met.  Sherry was an import, as well, except she was imported from Alabama to be a blind date for Hank.  As fate would have it, though, Sherry brought a girlfriend with her who also needed a date.  Hank hustled and found a friend named Rick to step in.  And "step in" he did, looking just like Robert Redford.  As soon as Sherry saw Rick, well, Hank didn't have a chance.  Poor guy.

It turned out to be a blessing, though, and another reminder that in the midst of a bruised ego, God wants us to trust in the bigger picture — and Hank's bigger picture consisted of me, yours truly, to complete him as a man.

The good news was Hank didn't have to wait too long before God rewarded him with me.  Of course, most folks in the Delta thought I was the one getting the prize.  I remember

Hank's sister, Jane Rule saying to me at least a dozen times on our wedding night, "Sallie, *you* are getting a prince. Never forget, *you* are getting a prince."

Sherry and Rick were married about a year before us and then they drove up to Memphis to witness Reverend Cheney administer our vows.   The four of us had become very close friends, along with Mary Ellen and her husband, Warren, who were married the following year.

Within nine years, we each had given birth to three babies.  Gosh, it still amazes me that we three imports cranked out nine little boys and girls with brand spanking new blood and DNA. What a gift to the Delta, don't ya think?

But, I know who has really been blessed.   When thinking of my children, I know without a doubt that my life puzzle is complete as long as Matt, Ben and Alden are a part of it.  There can be a zillion pieces missing and lost, but the love and mystery of these precious souls is simply enough.  Even so, my quest for "clarity, beauty and fulfillment" must continue – at least, if I'm going to finish this book!  And besides that, I still wanted a get-a-way!

### .... *Back to the get-a-way*

Sherry, Mary Ellen and I had taken to calling ourselves Thelma, Louise and Barbara — (don't ask). We had become a concrete triad of women built on trust, unconditional love and an amazing ability to make life a party when together.  So, it was a given that Sherry would have to go, too.

Funny, though, I had always assumed my first real get-a-way would be to the Golden Door Spa or something similar. You know, *relaxing.* But we were heading to the Big Apple — the city that never sleeps.

We realized the only real obstacle — after making arrangements for our children — would be convincing our husbands that the jaunt wouldn't cost too much.  With the hotel suite paid for, we quickly rounded up frequent flyer miles, companion passes, etc. and were able to afford our airline tickets.

All that was left was spending money!  Somehow, we figured we could do it for five hundred dollars each.  After all, we would barely be in New York for seventy-two hours.  Our husbands knew we were kidding ourselves, but softened anyway. Could it be they needed a break from us as well?  Nah.

So, as with all things planned spontaneously, we excitedly made our preparations.  I had not seen my two dear friends in months — in fact, not since my hysterectomy.

All of a sudden, I felt dowdy and thought a new outfit or two would help.  I immediately went to The Limited, where two teenage salesgirls helped me find just the right trendy attire for the trip.

On the day of our trip, I boarded my plane looking like

Petula Clark, in a mini leather skirt with go-go boots to match. I landed in LaGuardia Airport, only to find Mary Ellen and Sherry waiting for me...dressed in their usual style of casual elegance. They gave me the once over from head to toe, raised their eyebrows a bit, and then we erupted in laughter, joy and amazement that we really had pulled this off. And off we went to baggage claim; three grown women holding hands and giggling like little girls.

After realizing we had way too many bags for just one taxi, we were forced to hire a big, black, shiny limousine with a handsome uniformed driver to take us to our hotel. Oh well.

We asked him to put on some music, and then proceeded to dance, sing and boogie-on down Broadway. Our driver probably thought we were BORN in some little bitty town in Mississippi (not "imports" at all) — especially when I began to excitedly point out graffiti on the buildings.

After checking into our hotel, we immediately ordered room service. Three Coronas, two small bottled waters, a flower in a vase and a bill for sixty-seven dollars. "Uh-oh." We decided not to order water the next time.

The next few days were among the best of my life. We never stopped laughing, hardly slept and ate very little, as all we could afford was appetizers. Nevertheless, it was just what the doctor ordered for three stressed-out housewives and mothers. Not to mention a menopausal maniac.

My boots and bell-bottoms were a hit. Sherry was her naturally elegant, beautiful and classic self. Mary Ellen was her usual gorgeous and even *more* flamboyant self, and wherever we went, we turned heads. Or so we thought. Still, we enjoyed the ego feedback, whether it was real or not.

The first day we did Park Avenue, where everyone seemed rich and famous or at least employed by someone rich and famous. We had free makeovers, but of course bought lipstick just to be nice.

That night we went to see Smoky Joe's Café on Broadway and then practically closed down the LeBarre nightclub. We sat close to the band and became fast friends with the musicians on their breaks. We played Cupid with the female singer and the cute sax player who had been too shy to ask her out.

We counseled a gay guy on how to get his lover back who had jilted him that very day. "Play hard to get," we advised.

The three of us danced by ourselves and I accidentally backed into a guy and stomped on his foot. I turned to apologize and thought, "Oh, my, *it's Fabio.*" He smiled and said "No worry, it's a wooden leg." So much for Fabio.

We went to Soho and Greenwich the next day and rode the subway just for the experience. Some of our fellow passengers appeared a bit edgy; not to mention different so we rolled our diamond rings inside our palms and made Sherry tuck her emerald necklace inside her blouse just to be on the safe side.

As we were trying to figure out where and when to get off, the subway broke down. There we were, in utter darkness, under the streets of New Your City without a clue of what to do.

Thanks to the aid of the previously mentioned passengers, we finally found some stairs and ascended safely to the street above only to find ourselves in the heart of Times Square! The sun was just setting, the neon lights coming on and the gigantic Coca-Cola sign was flashing right in front of us. People, cars, taxis, and limos were buzzing around like crazy as the workday ended and the nightlife began. It was gorgeous—and almost overwhelming to our senses. We were finally speechless.

Upon arriving at our hotel, we hurriedly dressed to the hilt for our last night out. Mary Ellen in a backless black velvet halter gown, Sherry, 5'11", in a short black dress that made her legs look even longer than they were, and me? Well, I wore my old and faithful. Black velvet, strapless, floor length evening gown slit up to my upper thigh. Actually, when the dress was new, ten years before, the slit only went up to my knee. It had just ripped upwards an inch or two every time I wore it. Was it my lively dancing or my growing thighs?

My breasts are not as large or firm as they once were so I had to keep pulling my dress up at the top and down at the bottom to keep appropriately covered.

We tried to save the best for last, which we did — except for a few small sacrifices. We had reservations at The Four

Seasons for dinner, but bypassed that idea for lack of cash, only to find out the next day that Mary Ellen's father had called in his credit card for our unlimited use. Oops. But, we settled for champagne at The Oak Room in the Plaza instead and then rushed off to the theater to see *Phantom of the Opera.* We told the jolly man at the ticket booth how nice it was to see someone in New York smile. He responded by moving our seats about a hundred rows closer to the stage.

When we left the theater, still spellbound by the incredible play, we humbled ourselves-all dressed up, as we were, to begin hailing a taxi instead of a limo — to take us to our grand finale, The Rainbow Room. Mary Ellen and Sherry were taking pictures of each other under the Phantom signs and I, along with hundreds of others, began looking for transportation. All of a sudden, a white, l-o-n-g stretch limo pulled up and the driver whispered to me, "I'll take you anywhere for twenty-five dollars." *Wow,* I thought, *that's how much a taxi would cost.*

Now, I'm embarrassed to admit that I then pretended that the chauffeur and limo were OURS.

I yelled over to my friends, "Girls, come on! George is here."

Sherry and Mary Ellen looked at each other as if to say, *What in the world is she talking about?*

Then Mary Ellen yelled, "Who's George?"

I yelled back, "You know! GEORGE, our driver!"

By this time, the masses were watching us and the bad, prideful me thought, *Aren't we something, everyone thinks we're rich and famous.*

I finally got my friends to come over, and they kept mumbling about our lack of cash and not being able to afford a limo AND the Rainbow Room. But I kept up my charade, "Girls, come on! George has been waiting a long time."

The chauffeur was giving me weird looks, too. Of course, he was thinking, *Who the hell is George?*

Then I proceeded to open the door to get in. The problem was I couldn't find the door—*to my own limo!* Round and round it I walked, pulling the top of my dress up and the bottom part down. If the chauffeur hadn't gotten out of the driver's seat to show me the secret door, I would have never found it.

About this time, the police started yelling at the chauffeur to quit blocking traffic. So, I climbed in, ripping the slit in my dress another inch. Then, before Sherry and Mary Ellen could get in, the chauffeur closed the door and took off.

When he did, I lost my balance and hit my head on the television. I thought I was seeing stars but it was really the little white Christmas lights strung all over the ceiling of the limo. *Uh-oh,* I thought, *I'm in a pimpmobile!*

Before total panic overcame me, I heard screaming and saw Sherry and Mary Ellen, in their fine attire, running after the limo. "George" (his real name was Anthony, we found out later) finally stopped and let them in. *Whew.* I could feel a knot the size of a golf ball growing where I had hit my head, but at least my beloved friends were there.

The chauffeur lost his image as a pimp and became apologetic for having to leave the scene at the theater so fast. He said he couldn't afford to get another traffic ticket. We calmed down and then as we chatted in our southern accents, Anthony asked us where we were from. "Mississippi", we drawled.

He then told us his son was a football coach for a high school in a small town in Mississippi. It turned out to be the very high school our husbands had attended. In fact, it was the very town where our husbands were born and where Sherry and Mary Ellen still lived. Can you imagine? Of all the people and limos and taxi drivers, George (I mean Anthony) finds *us!* He treated us like queens after that, and for a few hours it was as if we really did own a limo and have a chauffeur all to ourselves.

He dropped us off at a special place outside the building on which the Rainbow Room was gloriously perched. Anthony assured us he would be waiting for us in a couple of hours. We noticed a long line of people waiting by some elevators as we went in, but before we knew it, some doormen were pointing us to other elevators and we were immediately taken to the top floor. As we exited the elevator, we saw another long line of people waiting to give their names to the maitre d'.

Mary Ellen whispered, "Follow me," which we obediently

did, right past the staring faces in line. She took us directly to the maitre d' table. Three handsome young Hispanic men in white tuxedos were manning the table and reservation book.

Mary Ellen proceeded to say, with her best Scarlett O'Hara tone, "Good evening, gentlemen. We don't have reservations, but we would appreciate a table as soon as possible *(pause — bat eyelashes)* with a view preferably."

They stood there gazing at us and looking a little concerned. Within seconds, an older man, obviously with more authority, arrived and quietly instructed them to give us table number twenty-one.

We were then whisked away to one of the best tables in the house. Sherry and I tried to act "normal" or should I say, "fake as fake can be," and Mary Ellen was acting like this was her normal way of life.

Guilt tried to invade my masquerade, but I pushed it away as I ordered a martini. Sherry ordered a Corona and Mary Ellen ordered — what else — champagne by the glass. We smiled as the three or four waiters hovered around us and opened the menus for us, but when they left, we freaked. There was a set price for just being there and the mere appetizers started at about thirty dollars.

We began figuring, with artificial smiles on our faces, "How in the world are we going to leave the Rainbow Room without washing dishes?"

During this time, the waiters kept coming over to refill Mary Ellen's champagne glass.

I finally touched one of their arms lightly, smiled and quietly asked, "How much are you charging her every time you refill her glass?"

"Twenty-four dollars, madam," he responded.

Obviously, she was cut off after that. Then the photographer comes over to take our photo. Just twenty bucks a piece. How could we refuse?

When our check for over four hundred dollars arrived, we managed to come up with the money and even found enough to tip our devoted waiters.

Sherry and I weren't too offended when one of the waiters asked Mary Ellen if she wanted to go up on the roof to see the skyline. After all, she was in her thirties, we in our forties. Plus her marriage was on the rocks.

Dear Anthony was indeed waiting for us when we left the Rainbow Room, but the glass partition was up. We were surprised when we heard a telephone ring. Mary Ellen found the phone and answered it. Of all people, it was Anthony.

He inquired, "What are you on?"

Mary Ellen thought for a minute, then began to point at each of us and say, "Well, she's on Prozac, and she's on estrogen and I'm on champagne.

Then he said, "No, I mean what street is your hotel on?"

After delivering us to our hotel, he promised to pick us up at seven o'clock in the morning, which was only four hours later. Somehow, we managed to pack up our scattered belongings, sleep three hours and make it down to the lobby.

I'll never forget the faces of my friends on the way to the airport. Such a contrast to the faces I had seen for the last two days. Of course, we were exhausted, not to mention starving and a bit hung over. But the despair and dread written all over Mary Ellen's face as she stared out the window was heartbreaking. Sherry also sat silently, with a scary sense of resignation that her own dilemma of blues would soon return. Her depression, though, like mine, was not so much circumstantial. It was of all things, "hormonal."

And me, I was exhausted, but okay. My *unplugging* process was becoming more tolerable, and I was looking forward to the peace and beauty of my home in the Sangre de Cristo Mountains. I was also excited to share my trip with Hank and the kids.

Funny, though, upon arriving home, the stress was greater than the biggest city in the country. The kids, naturally, were all over me, asking this and that. The worst part, though, was the silent resentment I sensed from Hank.

Was he insecure? Threatened? Worried? We did find out that as we were flying home, a lunatic with a machine gun massacred many people from atop the Empire State Building. And the fact that we never made it back to the hotel before three or four in the morning each night kept him awake wondering about our safety.

Nevertheless, his chilliness was evident, and it infuriated me. He had been on several hunting and fishing trips with the guys, not all of whom had good track records of being faithful to their wives. Besides, how could he feel insecure and threatened at this time in our lives when I loved him more than ever and my self-esteem was at its lowest? Maybe my love for him was being overshadowed by my low self-esteem. Perhaps he sensed danger, in that my unmet needs could possibly be met elsewhere.

Despair and the dark hole started creeping into my head and heart again. *"God, I just need some space sometimes. I feel like I'm suffocating. I'm sick of being all things to all people, of being accountable for everything I do. Even my kids stand ready to convict me at a moment's weakness. Don't I have a life anymore? I guess not."*

I was beginning to realize that my obsession to give life to another in my time of infertility was resulting in me losing my own life. My Christian self-help books even reminded me, "If you lose your life, you will find it." The authors also claimed that the serving of others would make me more Christ-like. Either they were wrong or I had a lot more serving to do.

*Fourteen*

## *The Grace of God*

**SILENCE**
*I need not shout my*
*faith.  Thrice eloquent*
*Are quiet trees and the*
*green listening sod;*
*Hushed are the stars*
*whose power is never spent;*
*The hills are mute: yet how they speak of God!*

— Charles Hanson Towne

*Spiritual* — a word so broad, yet narrow, a concept so
necessary to embrace, yet impossible to grasp a dimension that
encompasses the very essence of contrast.  My spirituality has
always evoked joy/sorrow, peace/conflict, guilt/comfort.

For years before my *unplugging*, I sought to find "the
peace that surpasses all human understanding."  I have just

recently begun to see that in my "seeking," I was blinded to the single most important ingredient of spiritual health — that of *grace*. I had heard, said and sung this word in a hundred songs, prayers and sermons, but I had never internalized the actual meaning of grace and all that it implies.

I simply missed the fact that there was absolutely nothing I could do to ensure God's love for me. This blunder set me up for years and years of fruitless effort. My inner emptiness rendered me vulnerable to just about what anyone was preaching. I am not proud of this feebleness on my part. In fact, I am ashamed that in my weakness I allowed myself to be abused, in a sense, by many theological disciplines.

## *Growing up*

As a child, I was a member of the Presbyterian Church in Miami Shores, Florida. My parents took their three children to Sunday school, church, choir and youth group every week. It was a ritual, a mandatory part of our lives that I don't remember ever questioning or complaining about. I also don't remember learning anything about God, except for the basics: the Christmas story, the Easter story, the Ten Commandments and the Apostles Creed.

I do, however, have vivid memories of certain events that took place at our church. My favorite ones include dressing up in a beautiful angel costume to participate in the huge, annual Christmas Nativity scene; sitting between my grandparents at church — Daddy-Milo, my grandfather, holding my hand, letting me play with his watch and grandmama letting me rub her long, smooth, cherry-red polished nails and my mother's beautiful voice loudly singing the hymns.

My not-so-favorite memories include my mother horrifyingly, for both of us, discovering I had shaved my legs when she patted my leg while sitting next to me in Church one Sunday; smoking pot for the first time on a youth church retreat and freaking out; getting married to the wrong guy in front of four hundred people; getting counseling from the minister who said after one session, "It is obvious your marriage has died. Now it is time to bury it," and the worst was the funeral of my dear Daddy-Milo. The family volunteered me to write and say a eulogy for him, which I did with voice shaking and tears streaming. It wasn't until after my speech that my brother told me I looked like a clown with way too much makeup on. How embarrassed I was and still am when I think of this. It has been sixteen years since my grandfather's death. Ridiculous, I know, but vanity has power — even in the midst of sorrow.

### Hearing with my heart

The first real testimony I received was from one of the

most popular "jocks" in my high school. He was a childhood friend, but I still held Jimmy in awe. One Sunday after church, he gave me a ride home and we stopped along the way at a favorite gathering spot we all called The Bay. The Bay was a special place on the Intracoastal Waterway, where I spent much of my childhood "playing" and much of my teen years "parking." A beautiful spot in Miami Shores where diving pelicans and zooming yachts entertained for hours and where the beauty of the Miami Beach skyline rendered people of all ages speechless.

I'll never forget that Sunday when Jimmy took me there and began witnessing to me. I actually "heard" with my heart for the first time the true message of the gospel. I remember being stunned as he told me I could have a one on one relationship with this "Jesus." I remember believing him, too — and then I went home and put this "Jesus" on the shelf — for somehow I thought He just may interfere with all the fun I was just beginning to have as a teenager.

Years later, just before Ron and I headed out on our six-month boat journey, a friend named Alice, from Birmingham, gave me the same testimony, so to speak. She told me that she had found something magical and wonderful that had changed her life. I'll never forget what she said: "Do you remember that place in the Bible where it says, 'Knock, and the door shall be opened' and 'Ask and you will receive'?"

I said, "Sort of," and she said, "Well, it works. Just try it and see what happens." Well, as you know, my life was a bit bleak at that time, so the next morning I went into the bathroom and knelt down on the floor to "knock," but I ended up using, for lack of a better analogy, a sledgehammer on the inner door of my soul. I begged and I pleaded, "God, if you're there, please hear me now." And then I began to wait for the life-changing magic Alice had said would be mine for the asking.

For the next few years, God did come into my life. Of course, I helped Him by reading the Bible and going to evangelical churches, where they taught me the concepts of "born again" and "saved." My bad habits didn't disappear right away, but I assumed God was just being gentle with me, as there was so much to change. Even so, I wondered what was taking God so long to turn my despair into happiness.

Many well-meaning fundamentalist Christian friends told me I was not being obedient enough or my faith was not strong enough. The only comfort I found was from a minister named Steve Brown, who would begin each sermon by saying, "Lord, we do not come to you because we are good, but because we are forgiven."

### Where and how to grow

When I married Hank, we immediately began to have problems about our preferences in churches. He would try to go to my more Bible-teaching church occasionally, yet his church always seemed to prevail as our regular place of worship. It was always a no-win situation, though. I eventually resigned myself to go to his church due to a pull towards submissiveness, and I also gave up hope Hank would ever leave the denomination he was born and raised in.

Hank loved the liturgy and communion we repeated every Sunday. He would kneel and read the same words as if they were different and more meaningful each week. I would kneel and try to concentrate on what I was saying, sometimes successfully, but mostly with unfounded resentment that these people and priests seemed not to worship with any spontaneity whatsoever. *Now, who was "judging" who?* I received helpful advice from an Episcopalian friend to focus more on what I could give to God instead of what He could give to me.

## *A miracle to behold*

I might not have straightened up and taken my one on one relationship with God so seriously if it were not for our second child, Ben, having been born fifteen weeks early, weighing 1 pound 15 ounces. I was barely halfway through my pregnancy when my body betrayed my baby by aborting him into the nightmare, roller-coaster world of prematurity.

After he survived his first two hours, he was transported

to a hospital in Jackson, Mississippi. When Ben had survived twenty-four hours, we rented an apartment in Jackson and moved there immediately. Ben remained in the hospital, in critical condition, for four months.

During that time, when Ben was at death's door, the neonatal doctors would say many times, "We've done all we can. If you believe in God, then start praying."

And pray we did, along with what seemed like the rest of the world. Ben was on prayer lists all over the country. Hank and I prayed for his life, for his comfort, for his eyesight and hearing — and hardest of all we succumbed once or twice to even pray for his death when we thought he was suffering needlessly at the hands of modern technology.

We went to a healing service every Friday at an Episcopal church down the road from the hospital. People would lay their hands on us as they prayed and I, again, mustered up my seed of faith in hopes of moving mountains.

One day as we were leaving the service, a little lady came up to us and told us that God had told her clearly that our son would not only live but would be completely normal. We returned to the hospital to find that Ben had made an amazing turnaround. His ventilator was taken out and the bleeding in his brain had vanished. Even the doctors were stunned. It was the first time in my life a miracle occurred before my eyes. Many more miracles would astound both Hank and me, but the doctors were especially amazed as Ben overcame impossible odds.

I began to visualize little angels (like Tinkerbells) buzzing gently around Ben. I saw them healing him within and comforting him from the pain, bright lights and bedlam of the neonatal unit. Was I seeing things? I don't know, but Ben left that hospital weighing three and a half pounds and is now fourteen years old and perfectly wonderful.

### *"Settling"*

I joined a non-denominational charismatic women's prayer group when we returned to Greenville in order to supplement the dryness I felt in Hank's church. These ladies told me I did not have the gift of the Holy Spirit because I did not speak in tongues. So one day I knelt in the middle of a lady's living room and they all gathered around me, placed their hands on my head, began speaking in their tongues and anointed me. I tried to utter some sounds and as I did, they all "praised the Lord," but that was all that ever happened. I never went back. I assumed my faith was not strong enough for the Holy Spirit to bestow a foreign language on me.

I finally relented and accepted that Hank's church would have to do. I even agreed to join a special study program the church offered. One of the past graduates of the program was assigned to be my partner. In my newfound humility, God shined through and gave me a beautiful older woman named Sue to be my partner. She met with me weekly and eventually became more than a partner. She became my counselor, my friend, and my saving grace. Her open-mindedness, her loving and accepting spirit, and her wisdom began the long sought-after unfolding of my own spirituality.

### *Letting others stunt our growth*

Unfortunately, my spiritual renewal was short lived. We moved to Colorado soon after and bought a house in town, where we would live until we were ready to begin construction on the land we had purchased in the mountains. We lived there for a year until we decided to sell the house for an offer we would be foolish not to accept. During that year, I tried to maintain my spiritual vigor by befriending some local Christians, only to find out that they too were putting God in a little judgmental box.

For instance, my neighbor at the time, a beautiful girl who resembled Jane Seymour, was utterly convinced that only four hundred people were really the bride of Christ and they would be the ONLY souls allowed into heaven upon the second coming of Christ. If I confronted her with a differing interpretation, she became fiercely defensive. Needless to say, our friendship withered away about as quickly as it began.

Of course, the timing could not have been worse as I had

just been attacked by "instant menopause." Somehow, my Jane Seymour look-alike became the straw that broke my *holy* camel's back.

I began doubting everything I had ever believed. I didn't exactly become an atheist, since all I had to do was look at Ben to remember my proof.

Nevertheless, my days of judging and using "born again" lingo were over. I accepted that I didn't know it all after all, and then I allowed apathy to set in. I was still a "believer," but I felt no need to be a fisher of men or even a churchgoer and decided that the English language worked quite well as a God-given tongue.

As the closing date of our house grew near, it became evident that we were not going to find an available house to rent while our new home was under construction. Somehow, in my menopausal state, I let Hank talk me into moving into a motor home. He hooked it up to the building site's septic and electrical and assured me we would be in the house within a few weeks. Hah! A soon-to-be *unplugged* woman living in a very *plugged-in* motor home.

Hank, myself, three children, four dogs, two birds and a cat lived in that thing for close to four months in the dead of winter. Hank put a big tent up behind the motor home and named it the "sanity tent." I thought it was set up for my sanity; only to find out it was for HIS sanity when my *insanity* flared up.

No wonder that same 'ol dark hole kept trying to vacuum

me up. Maybe it had nothing to do with hormones. Maybe it was just the darn motor home.

Nevertheless, it was an experience I *think* I am glad happened. I could kneel down in the middle of the kitchen floor and spray Fantastic 360 degrees and with two paper towels clean the entire floor in two minutes.

We had packed and stored everything we owned, except for some shirts and jeans, and enjoyed the revelation that simplicity was possible. Even so, we gratefully *unplugged* and moved into our new home as soon as we had any semblance of plumbing and enough visqueen to keep us somewhat free of plaster and sawdust.

### And along came an angel

It was about this time that a messenger came to me in the form of a homeless woman named Suzanne. She and her mate, Jerry, our tile-layer, pulled their own mobile home, an old van, up to our house each day while Jerry worked on our house.

Suzanne would sit in that van most of the day crocheting, studying, and meditating. Once or twice, she would take a brief walk or just sit outside. She was about fifty years old and everyday she would wear a different hippie-type dress, skirt or blouse made of Indian cotton with beautiful prints and patterns.

As I would come and go from my home, we would speak

briefly to one another. I felt guilty and intimidated that we were building such a fine home when they lived in a van. What could we ever have in common? And worse, what if they asked to temporarily share our unfinished house. The selfish, uncompassionate part of me was hesitant to give this strange woman an inch for fear that they might take a mile. Would they then ask to move in with us and never leave?

After they had been at the house for about a week, I came down with an awful case of the flu. Jerry told Suzanne that I was ill and she asked Hank if she could come in to visit with me for a few moments. What could he say? What could I say?

She came in and sat with me, in the one room free of sawdust and plaster. She spoke of herbs that might help me get well and then asked what spiritual *"path"* was I on. *Here we go again,* I thought. *Another laying on of the hands, then the testimony and so on.*

I told her I wasn't really on a path anymore. That I was basically a Christian, but I was at a stopping point growth-wise due to the "God in the box" mentality.

*Well, let's have it,* I thought, *give me your spiel and then please leave.*

I politely said, "I'm really very tired, but quickly tell me what 'path' you are on."

She said, "Well, I'm personally on the Christian path, but

Jerry follows Native American traditions and rituals. I also have many friends on the Hindu path. But, we are one in that we are all heading to the same God."

*Wow,* I thought, *this is interesting. An open-minded Christian.* I knew my fundamentalist friends would say this is new age theology sent to me from the devil.

"Tell me more," the rebellious side of me said. I was suddenly not so eager for her to leave.

She told me that she and Jerry were "earth travelers" and that they chose to live in the van so they could always be mobile to minister to people whose paths they crossed. She talked about the homeless and how their numbers would be increasing as the future of our planet changed. These were the people they especially felt called to help.

And there she was helping *me*, a bit homeless myself. It suddenly seemed like no coincidence that our physical *and* spiritual paths had crossed.

Upon leaving she said, "Sallie, it is important for you to know that apathy is an enemy to you — especially spiritually."

### Another call to fitness

Suzanne's words stayed with me as I slowly recovered from the flu. I realized she was right about apathy. It is an enemy. Passiveness leads to a state of atrophy, similar to what lack of exercise does to our bodies. Staying spiritually fit suddenly seemed of great importance to me.

In my reasonably *unplugged* state, I began to contemplate accepting all paths to the Father, the Truth or the Divine. I began "knocking and seeking" again. But this time I listened not so much to others, but to my heart. And in so doing, I heard the path of Christianity calling me back. I heard the words of Jesus saying, "Come unto me." These were the words He said to His disciples two thousand years ago. These were the words carved on the statue of Jesus under the sea, which first brought Hank and me together.

Yes, I returned to the God of my childhood, but humbled and comforted by the mystery of faith. I had found a new appreciation for the uniqueness and individuality of the spirituality of others, even within the same denomination. My humility came from the realization that I had generalized, stereotyped and judged the very people who I assumed were judging me.

Paula D'arcy articulated my feelings in her beautiful book, *Gift of the Red Bird.* She said:

> " I read about God as masculine. God as feminine. God speaking boldly. God in the stillness. God seemed to change or move each time I decided I understood, too securely, who He was. Increasingly, I saw the holy in the ordinary and the sacredness of all creation. The love of God raced ahead of me, and I could hardly take in its depth and breadth."

My new open-minded theology has not pleased some of my

friends. In fact, a few have told me that I have been deceived by the devil. My children have even been accused of not being "Christians" because they do not attend the local Evangelical Church. How angry this must make our heavenly Father — when the pure and simple faith of children is put before the courts, the judges, and the juries of man.

The good news is that in spite of trials and tribulations, our family continues to live and grow. We are surrounded by mountains, forests, summer wildflowers and winter snow. Our skies are periwinkle by day and star-studded by night. God is truly present in our lives.

We have lost loved ones to death, yet we know their spirits go on. My little girl, Alden, even names a star after each family member, friend or pet we have had to bury. She'll say, "Look, Mommy! There's Judy or there's Dane or there's Stardust (our colt) and Stony (our cat) and Lacey (our dog).

Hank and I teach our children that there is light and dark, good and evil, and that they must choose accordingly. We have told them that we, their parents, believe that God made himself into a human being named Jesus Christ so He would know our struggles on this earth. We celebrate His birth, His death and His resurrection. Yet we do not judge the beliefs of other people.

## *Tolerance, Truth and Trust*

This *unplugging* from the traditional rules and regulations of organized religion has been a slow yet wonderfully liberating journey for me. The best part is to see that my open heart is enabling me to love more and hate less, which has great rippling effects. We have no idea what makes people tick, what issues they have had to live with, or what DNA makeup they have inherited.

One of my favorite songs is called "At The Same Time" by Barbara Streisand on her *Higher Ground* album. Some of the words are:

*Think of all the hearts beating in the world — at the same time*
*Think of all the faces and the stories they could tell — at the same time*
*Think of all the eyes looking out into this world*
*Trying to make some sense of what they see*
*Think of all the ways we have of seeing*
*Think of all the ways there are of being*
*Yes, think of all the hearts beating in this world — at the same time*

This is the message I wish to pass on to my children and others — to love everyone. It's not about taking on their lifestyle as your own or denying your own sense of values. It is just about acceptance and compassion. These character traits are contagious. They will first pass from us to our families and then to one generation after another. I truly believe, as a result, there will be less hate and fear in the world and most certainly, more joy and peace in our hearts.

I see now that in all the years I allowed myself to be influenced by this or that person or philosophy, I was missing the most important point. I was "seeking," but not "seeing." I was "knocking," but not opening the door. God's presence was there and always has been. It was just veiled under my preoccupation with performance, pride and people pleasing.

I also missed along the way that one doesn't earn a relationship with God. If we are truly created in His image, and if indeed, His Holy Spirit resides within us, then we are one with God, one with one another, one with all of nature — connected eternally.

This precious alliance comes to us free of a price, at least on our part as Christians. Jesus of Nazareth paid our price in full so that we may keep our humanity and still have access to, not only God's eternal kingdom, but to His protection and guidance on earth in the here and now. All that is required of us is faith that this man named Jesus is truly God's son. A pretty easy task for even a skeptic. All one needs to do is look at the truth, which has been staring back at us for centuries.

If this man was a myth, then why does the human race date their timelines, from present to future with time B.C. and time A.D.? And why does the world continue to acknowledge the birth of this man, the death of this man, the resurrection of this man whether it is with sincere hearts or commercial enthusiasm?

And how is it possible that there is more proof that Jesus Christ walked and lived than there is of Julius Caesar?

Many of my friends do not acknowledge a supreme being, but prefer to pray to the Universe or to a higher power within themselves.  I somehow need to know the origin or source of my higher power in order to really count on it.  Like who or what will charge our batteries when the inevitable burdens of life become too much to bear.

Does a vast generator in the sky simply kick on and replenish our higher power — even in the tragic midst of losing a child, of being diagnosed with cancer, or any number of other shattered dreams?

Or, do we call on our CREATOR, our SOURCE, our CONNECTION?  This is when our lives are so full of darkness and chaos — that just knowing there is a light somewhere may get us through.

Another of my favorite authors is Madeleine L'Engle.  In one of her Crosswicks Journal Series called *A Circle of Quiet,* L'Engle shares with her students what she believes are the three ways you can live your life:

First, she says, "You can live life as though it's all a cosmic accident; we're nothing but an irritating skin disease on the face of the earth."

Or secondly, she says, "you can go out at night and look at the stars and think, 'yes', they were created by a prime mover and so were you, but this force is aloof to perfection, impassible, and indifferent to creation. You don't matter, and I don't matter, except possibly as a means to an end."

"Or thirdly," she says, "you can live as though you believe that the power behind the universe is a personal power of love, a love so great that all of us really *do* matter. In fact, our creator loves us so much that every single one of our lives has meaning; And the fall of every sparrow is indeed acknowledged."

Madeleine L'Engle picks the last scenario to base her faith upon. I'm with her.

*Fifteen*

# *Jack of NO Trades*

With my spiritual fitness renewed, I began to walk forward in life, menopause and all — confident that my chosen path would soon lead me into peace and prosperity.  Okay, maybe not prosperity, but peace combined with a sense of purpose.  This was my quest.

My lack of purpose has always been an underlying virus in my life that would surface every now and then, like a rash.  But my imaginary virus turned into a chronic obsession, more like the hives, when I was thrown into menopause so abruptly.

It seems as if all of my life I have been praying and waiting for a special gift, talent, or calling I could center my life around. Why? I don't know. Is this a common desire most people have? I've known many people who seem content to just "be," and at times I thought I had become one of them.

With contentment, I would go weeks and sometimes months with little, if any, inner pressure to accomplish more than living successfully in the present. All the while, I would be enjoying the moments of life, the spontaneity — just cruising along with a sense of contentment. Granted, it was a lovely and worthwhile way to live, but not practically possible, at least for me.

The problem was my satisfaction with just "being" was short-lived. My desire to "do" always returned. It took me a while to understand that "being" and "doing" is a balancing act. Both are crucial to the success of each. For instance, my writing would come quickly to a standstill if I did not take time to smell the roses every now and then. On the other hand, if I had no meaningful work or special project awaiting me, the carefree passing of days would eventually leave me restless.

Nevertheless, in my menopausal struggle, I was not aware of the necessity of balancing *being* with *doing*. I was only aware of that familiar void. I needed a purpose or a mission that would give me a reason to be here. Something that would justify my existence. Sad, but true.

I hoped this singular focus would also profit me financially, as well as emotionally. And, when my days on earth were finished, I hoped my life would have made a difference on this earth. Hah! The new midlife cynic in me shouted, "baloney!" I became almost resigned to believe that there was no strength, purpose, or talent

*"After becoming umbilically unplugged, we remain free of expectations and pressures, and most of us live our lives as carefree children."*

Top right: Me in the first year of my life. Top left: Me with my daddy, Uncle Ted and Uncle Jimmy. Bottom: My "Leave it to Beaver" family (from the left) me, my mom, my sister, dad and brother.

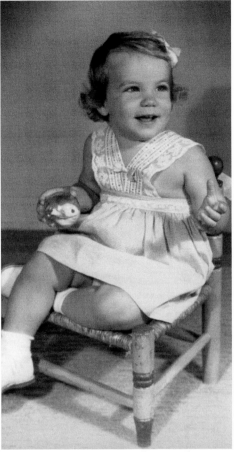

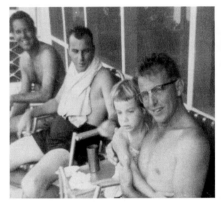

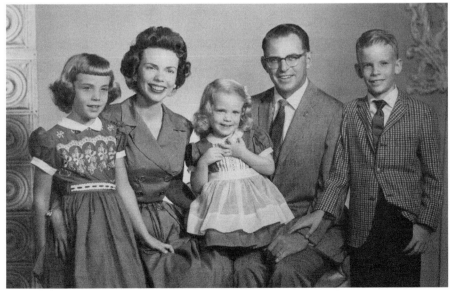

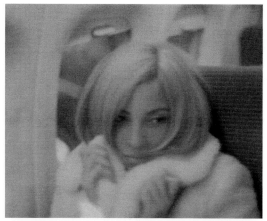

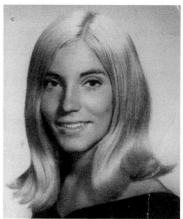

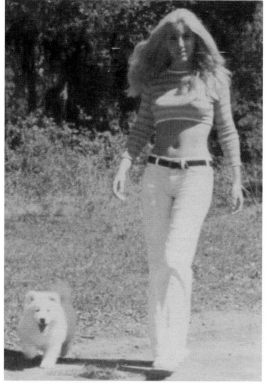

*"The onset of puberty, however, begins our own experience of increasingly becoming plugged-in."*

Top left: Taking off after Charm School, scared and not quite ready for what was expected of me.

Top right: Who is *that* girl?

Middle: A Barbie-Doll rendition of me...still a stranger to myself.

Bottom left: From Daddy to Delta....*Finally* my daddy seems proud of me.

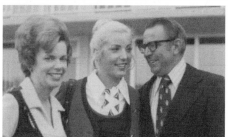

# *Headlines! Culture shock!*

Two worlds collide!…. Miami Beach, 3$^{rd}$ generation native, Sallie Astor marries "most eligible" Mississippi Delta Gentleman, Hank Burdine whose roots outlive those of his bride.

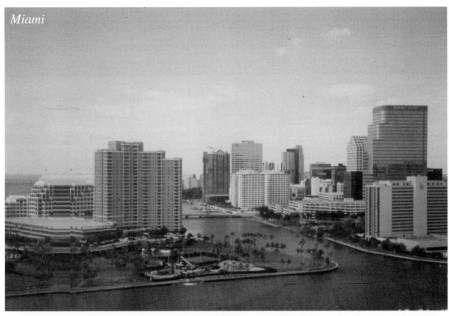

*Miami*

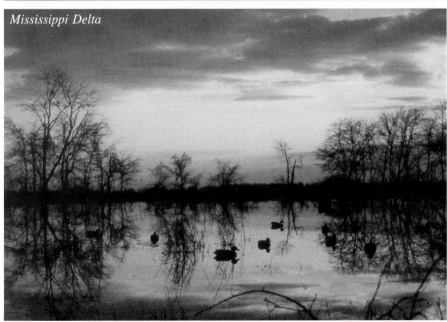

*Mississippi Delta*

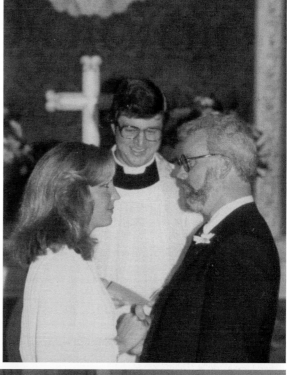

### *Wedding bells, babies and big dreams come true...*

Top: Hank and I saying our wedding vows.

Bottom: Our wedding night.

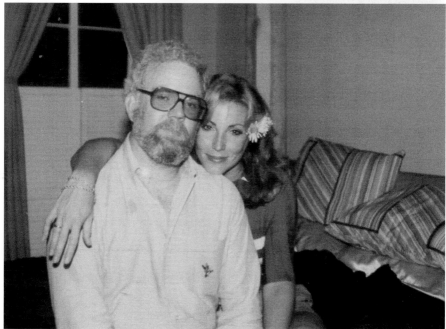

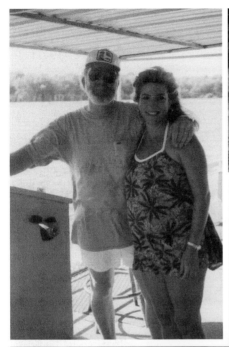

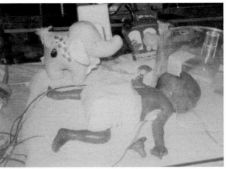

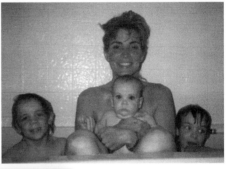

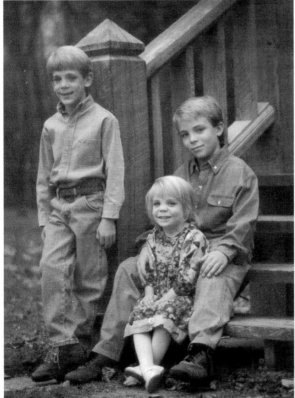

Top left: Pregnant...at last!

Top right: Our miracle baby, Ben.

Middle right: Scrub-a-dub-dub, three babies (and a Mama) in a tub.

Bottom left: Picture Perfect.

Top:  Baby Jane Burdine and Jane Astor meet their grandson, Ben.

Bottom: Mary Ellen and I introduce our first borns, Catharine and Matthew, who, like their moms, would be future soul mates.

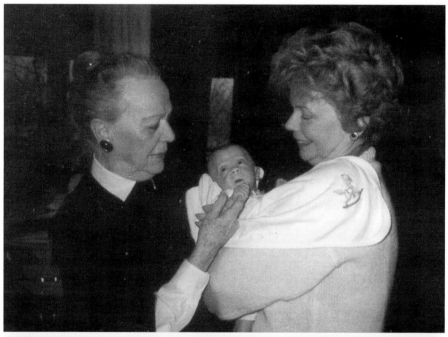

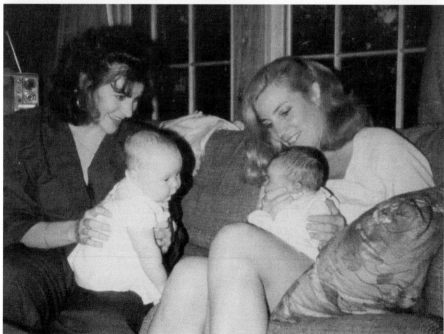

## *The imports growing babies, seemingly everywhere you turn.*

Top (left to right): 32 years old and finally complete, (or so I thought!)...the happiest time in my life. Sherry sits next to me pregnant with Sarah as her son, Will, pats her tummy.

Bottom (left to right in the back): Will Smythe, Catharine Hammet, Sarah Smythe. (left to right in the front): Ben Burdine, and Matt Burdine. Five of the nine children, Mary Ellen, Sherry and I (three each) contributed to the gene pool of the Delta...enjoying a day on the mighty Mississippi River.

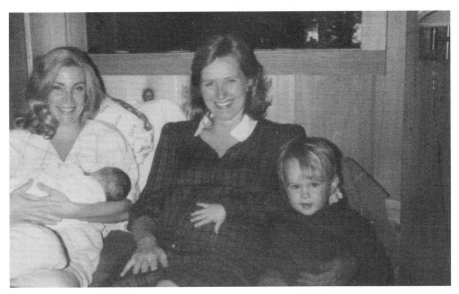

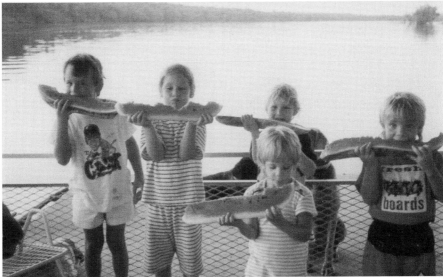

# *A handful and a heartful...*

*Matt, our first, Ben, our miracle,
and Princess Alden.*

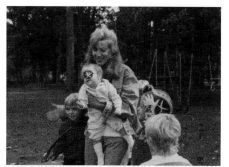

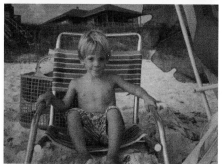

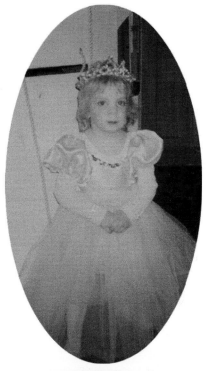

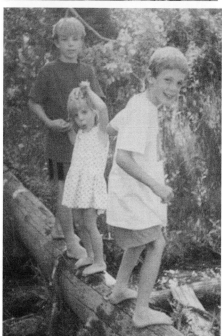

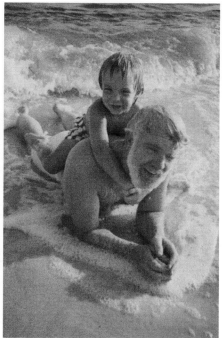

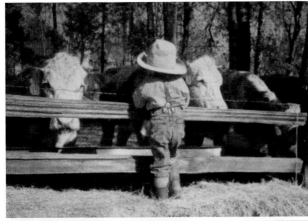

*...yet, still seeking purpose and meaning...still justifying my existence.*

Top: Breeding registered Polled Hereford cattle.

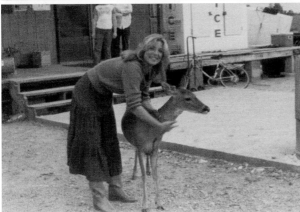

Middle: Animal Welfare Activist.

Bottom: Practicing for a trap shooting competition.

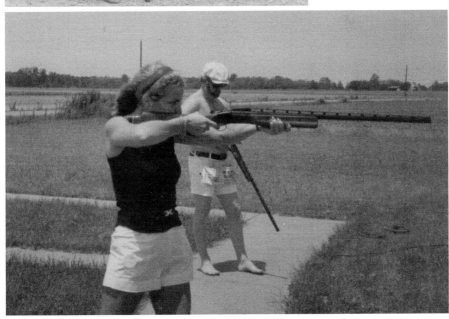

## *Escape to New York City*

Top right: Sherry and Sallie decked-out for a night on the town.

Top left: Mary Ellen and Sherry enjoying "George's" limo.

Bottom: Country gals come to town.

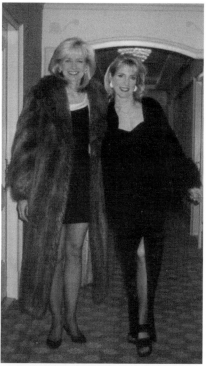

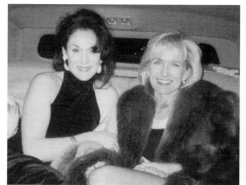

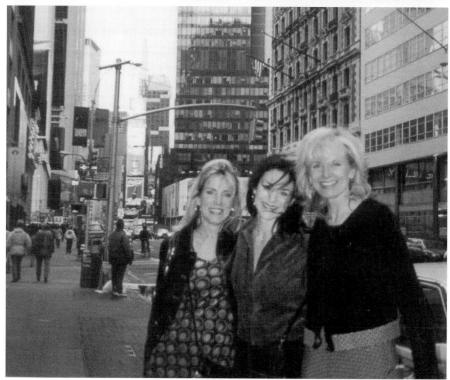

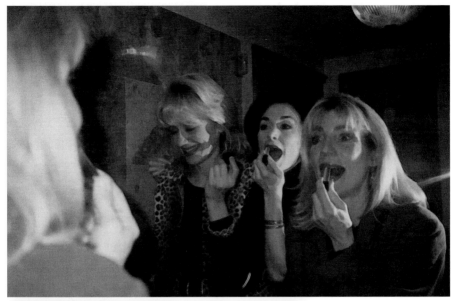

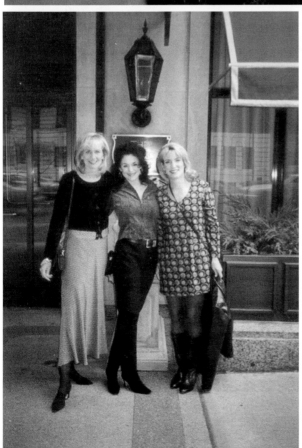

### ....*New York City continued*

Top: Primping after lunch.

Bottom: Thelma, Louise and Petula Clark look-a-like —*yours truly*.

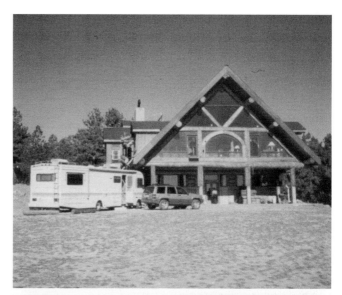

## *Midlife and motor-home madness*

Top: *Very plugged-in* to the motor home.

Bottom: *"Contemplation."*

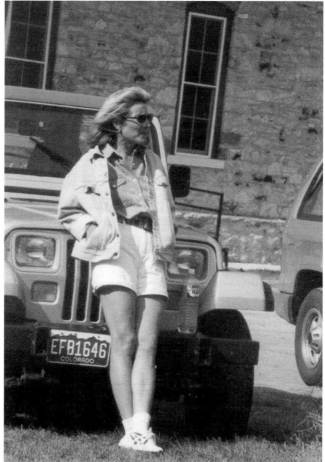

140

## *Phantom Canyon Detour*

Top left: Mary Ellen and I raring to go (we usually don't match...promise).

Top right: Maya, our epileptic canine passenger, with Audrey...her owner and my dear friend.

Bottom: Finally home safe and sound.

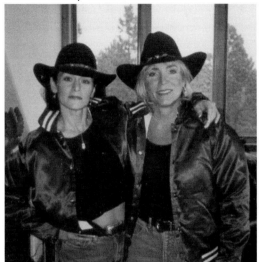
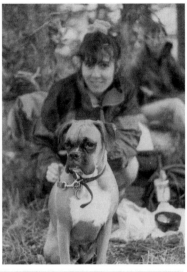
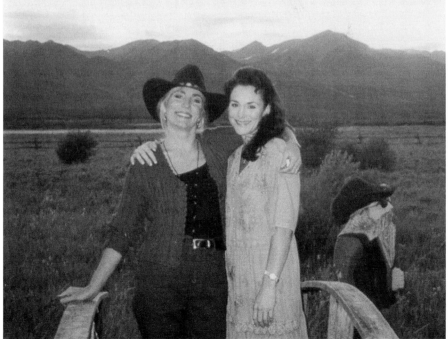

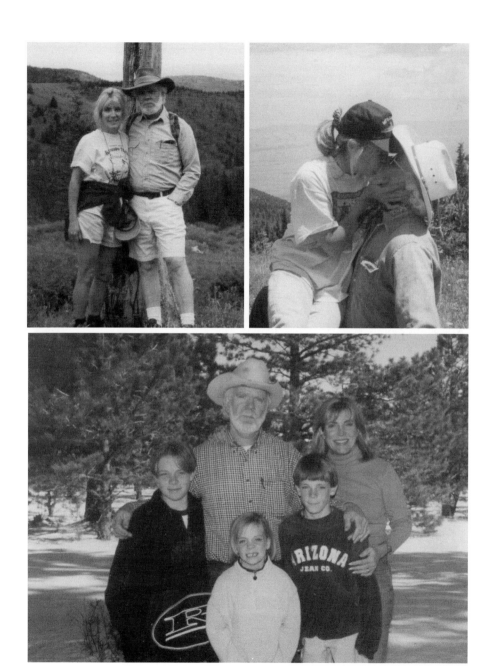

Top left and right: Hank and me...finding ourselves in each other.

Bottom: A family of five.

*Unplugged...*

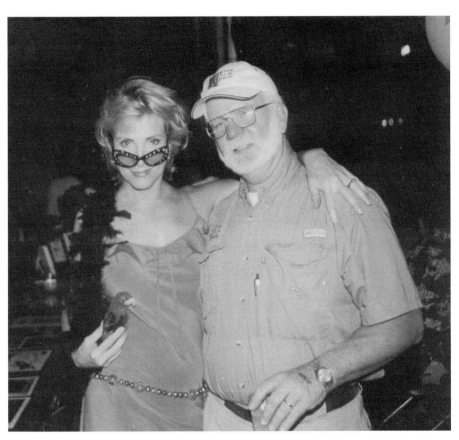

Hank and me *unplugging* galore on our 19th wedding anniversary.

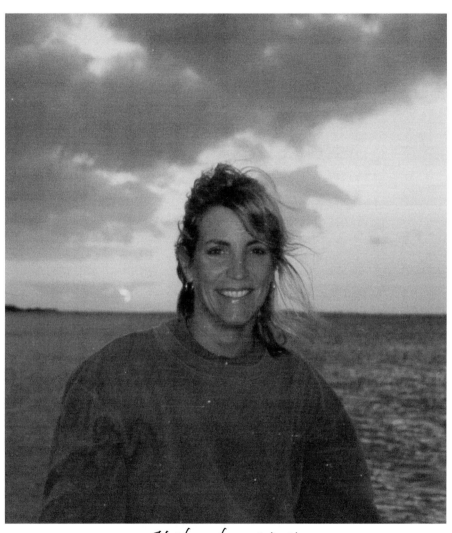

*Unplugged...* at last!

in me.

The saying "jack of all trades, master of none" used to drive me mad, in that I coveted this description whereas most people resented it. I was a classic "jack of NO trades," much less a "master of anything!"

Do I sound arrogant for resenting my lack of having an obvious gift or great reason for being here? Maybe so, but a life without meaning or direction seems too painful for me to bear. Perhaps that is why this issue was such a difficult one for me to tackle when it became obvious that the first half of my life was over.

Just like an irritating ulcer in one's mouth, my lack of purpose became a constant reminder that something was missing. Sometimes tolerable, sometimes painful, but the void was nevertheless always there.

In looking back, I can see that the hope for meaning has always been there. I always had a certain sense of confidence that my true self would surface and all would be well. I just knew that one-day when someone asked, "And what do YOU do?", I would be able say, "I'm a psychologist" or "I'm a potter" or "I'm a dog breeder." And there have been many times when I have had an answer of which I was proud. The problem was that the answer changed every few months or weeks or even days.

Once I was able to say, "I'm an animal welfare activist." I went around to schools with my slide show on how to feed and care for pets. I preached the importance of spaying and neuter-ing. I even "saved the whales" and crusaded against animal ex-perimentation.

When I married a "hunter," I became a vegetarian to escape being labeled a hypocrite. My friend, Fidelia, taught me to say, "I don't eat anything with a face." My ethics were honor-able, but my ignorance about combining proteins eventually cost me a month in bed.

My next lesson was learning to see the color gray when it came to the tough issues of life. For instance, if a poor little mouse had not been experimented on, my laser brain surgery to remove a pituitary tumor would have left me bald and blind.

I once decided to breed prized polled Hereford cattle. Just imagine...a vegetarian turned cattle breeder. And to think we used artificial insemination. My husband's secretary almost fainted when UPS delivered a silver smoking cylinder containing frozen semen from a famous bull named Enforcer. The funny part was that Enforcer had been dead for five years. The sad part was all the money my husband lost when my interest in cows faded.

The trapshooting obsession came next, complete with a new Remington shotgun and a wardrobe to match. Pregnancy ended that venture for fear my baby would be traumatized, if not deafened, from the blasting guns.

While my children were being born and raised into

toddlerhood, I succumbed to a quick but intense bout with what I call "multi-level mania." It was the perfect solution to my lack of "doing" (what in the world did I think having three children under the age of five was?)

This "multi-level mania" opportunity seized me with what all the propaganda intended it to do. Not only would my family be blessed with riches beyond dreams, but I would help others climb out of their ruts and teach them to help others as well. I managed to reach the sapphire (or was it ruby?) level, but needless to say, this venture belly-flopped and left me with a nice dose of humility and regret, not to mention a warehouse full of products.

Soon after, I bought the fitness center with the inheritance my grandfather left me. Again, I was going to help people and profit financially from it as well. Again, my intentions were honorable, but my expertise was lacking. I kept the center for about a year until I decided that owning a health spa was hazardous to my health because I never had time to exercise, not to mention that I was selling addictive herbs.

Next came the national franchise chain I decided to start from scratch. It was going to be good, healthy fast food that was low in fat and delicious. "Hearty, yet heart-wise." A simple undertaking. My ever-supportive husband hired me an accountant, a chef to create our menu and even gave me full access to his brilliant bookkeeper. And the rest is history, not to mention a nice tax deduction due to capital loss.

It still amazes me that I was truly optimistic about ALL of these ventures. When something grabs me, it consumes me. None can surpass my enthusiasm, at least in the startup phase, anyway.

I do realize that my children have given and continue to give me a huge sense of purpose. When they were little, my days were filled with loving and caring for them. Three little ones in five years was definitely a handful. They were, and still are, also a heart-full.

The births of each of our children were not without major difficulties. It was after four long and trying years of infertility that we were finally able to conceive our firstborn, Matt. Six months later, we were with child again, only our second son, Ben, decided to escape my womb halfway through the pregnancy.

After two miscarriages, our daughter, Alden, was born by cesarean. Did I mention that I had to stay in bed for seven months prior to her birth?

You see, nothing of real value has ever come easy for me, but it always comes sooner or later, if I try hard enough. Maybe that's why my sense of hope and confidence has always been there.

With my motherhood established and maternal instincts satisfied, I felt a certain blissful sense of completion. At least, until the kids started attending school all day — right on the heels of my emergency hysterectomy. Without knowing it, I was being faced with my first *unplugging* of previous roles and it stung.

Seemingly overnight, I was faced with just myself again and the old questions of purpose and meaning began to haunt me. It wasn't "empty nest" syndrome; I was relieved to have my life back. And even though the children may have slipped from my arms, their dirty clothes and constant clutter kept my arms full all day long. The sheer routine of daily chores and endlessly repetitive housework can drive the best of homemakers crazy, to say the least.

One day, I caught myself thinking, *"It has come to this now. I am literally in the middle of my life. The growing-up period has ended and the growing old period is beginning. I am on top of the mountain, and now my choice is to climb back down or pick another mountain."*

The optimist in me shouted, *Climb! Climb! Keep climbing!* But the realist in me knew that gravity would eventually win (at least in some areas, like my breasts and rear-end).

Then the optimist responded, *Gravity can be slowed down, but wisdom, peace and joy can be accelerated.*

So I picked another mountain and hoped the hike up might firm up my tush as well as enrich my soul. With the decision made to keep growing instead of slowly rotting, the conflict returned.

*Which mountain? And which trail would insure that the*

*journey would be as rewarding as the destination?*

I once heard that destiny can have many voices, but we still must make choices. It is those voices and choices that frustrated me before and during the crossing. Little did I know that every choice I ever made was what had brought me to exactly where I needed to be today. All the frustration and pressure I put upon myself was for naught. Every choice and every consequence prepared me to find purpose on the other side of midlife madness.

In *Your Life as Story,* Tristine Rainer writes of her own quest to make sense of her fragmented life. At the age of forty, she realized she had done many different jobs and none of them were indicative of a particular career progression. But after looking more closely at her list of past jobs, she was delighted to find a thread of continuity in her life. All of her past jobs showed a definite interest in learning about people's individual stories.

It was Rainer's book that helped me look at the scattered pieces of my own life and see the connection between most of my ventures. The animal welfare activist, the multi-level mania, the health food chain and the fitness center all show I wanted to help people find a better way. Whether it be by showing them compassion for animals, themselves and others, by getting them out of a financial rut, or by helping them become healthier. I was amazed and relieved to find some continuity — any continuity —

in this vastly interrupted life of mine.

I am convinced that human beings have an innate need to give something back to the world in which we live — whether it's from a sense of obligation to contribute or merely the physical manifestation of a creative power they possess. I believe our authenticity, our becoming *real*, depends on our tuning in, so to speak, to our special gift.

Unfortunately, before we can ever begin to plug-in, much less unplug — we are stifled and distracted enough to easily take the wrong road.

Think of a small child drawing a masterpiece on a wall, building a castle or fort with blocks, singing and pretending. And then watch the creativity that was once natural and free dwindle for most children as they grow into teens and then adults.

I imagine that as children, our creativity is diminished by criticism and a lack of self confidence. Then, as teens and young adults, the practicality of life becomes the priority. We have to go to school, join clubs, participate in sports. Plug in.

Next, as adults, we are faced with financial and other responsibilities that rob us of the time and energy to even explore, much less develop our creative side.

The result is that many of us must settle for a job that we resent, but feel is the financially responsible thing to do. Granted, there are many cases where people have no choice. But there are probably just as many cases where courage and persistence could remedy a life eaten up by an unpleasant job or a *senseless* sense of duty.

I have wasted much of my life carelessly taking on extra burdens of responsibility. Many times, I have accepted positions on committees or volunteered my efforts on projects that were of little importance to me. Maybe I felt too guilty to say no or maybe I looked forward to the credit I would receive. Who knows?

But accepting responsibilities for the wrong motives in the wrong areas happens when we haven't identified what is really important to us. Of course, experiencing assorted areas of work is not what stifles and exhausts us. It is *remaining* in a situation that doesn't suit us that is the true detriment to our growth and eventual fulfillment.

*Sixteen*

# *Jack of ONE Trade*

In my longing to find a niche, a direction, a purpose, I went from impulse to impulse until I hit the right one for me — writing. Who would have thought it? It has been close to six years now since I began writing, and my computer and notebook continue to draw me like a magnet.

My husband actually came up with the idea that I begin a book. We were driving back to Mississippi from Colorado for a visit and I was venting my menopausal obsession to him about what to do with the rest of my life.

He simply said, "Write a book about it."

I said, "A book? What about?"

He said, "About everything. Write your story with its ups and downs and share your frustrations and all that you've learned."

I said, "I think I will."

At the next gas stop, I bought a loose-leaf notebook and began going backwards from my new midlife crazies — listing issues along the way — and before I knew it, I was a little girl again.

I started out like a whirlwind, similar to my other endeavors, but knowing and fearing that this too could end up as "another one bites the dust." Hesitantly, I began telling my closest friends and family what I was up to — knowing that many of them were probably laughing at Sallie's newest venture. After all, my track record was not exactly great in the completion department.

Nevertheless, I began to write. Feelings, memories, whatever came to mind at first. I was computer illiterate, but I figured out how to open and save a document and began typing. I was also literary illiterate, in that I had never had a course in creative writing, my grammar was dubious, to say the least, and basically, I had no clue as to how to write a story, much less a book. But I became obsessed with finding out. I went to the library and the bookstores and brought home books on every facet of writing and the publishing world.

And then, in keeping with the synchronicity of life (no coincidences), a writing workshop was advertised in our local newspaper. A distinguished writing teacher, Ferris Frost, was coming to our little town of six hundred to spend a day with writer wannabes. I signed right up. As I sat there with about twenty other participants, I became acutely aware that I was starting at zero in ability. But, for what it was worth, I was starting at one hundred in terms of desire and interest.

A week after the workshop, I contacted Ferris at her office and asked her if she would be interested in taking a look at what I had written so far. She was kind enough to say yes, and I started faxing her sheets and sheets of single spaced, wordy and confusing pieces of paper, in tiny eight-point font to boot. She would send them back to me with encouraging comments like "Keep writing!" and "Go for it!" along with bits and pieces of constructive criticism on every line in red ink. She also said with great gentleness that I had no structure, no direction and was contradicting myself chronologically at every turn. *No kidding,* I thought, *my writing is just like my life!*

Eventually, thanks to Ferris's encouragement, I discovered how to apply some structure to my work and, just as important, I learned how to enlarge the type size on my computer so that she could read what I had written without a magnifying glass.

I was also fortunate to have a dear friend who is an acclaimed Southern writer, Bern Keating. He also began to read my output and patiently taught me that I had much to learn. He immediately assigned Strunk & White's, *Elements of Style* and Zinsser's, *on Writing Well* as required reading for me. Through these books and his own expertise, Bern taught me the importance of saying something more powerfully with eight words instead of eighteen. This is obviously a process I am still working on, so bear with me.

It still amazes me that these two professional and well-educated authors did not resent my naiveté in thinking I could write a book so easily. Instead, they encouraged, constructively criticized, and encouraged again and again. I will be forever grateful to them.

For the next six months, my goal was to prepare and send out book proposals to as many publishing houses as seemed compatible with my book.

I achieved my goal and sent out approximately forty proposals. And then I waited. Within several weeks, I received about twenty rejections that looked like form letters, most of which said they do not accept unsolicited manuscripts. Another ten or so came as personal notes. Most were encouraging but nevertheless were rejections. I have not heard from the rest and assume my proposal ended up in the slush piles, along with thousands of other unread manuscripts.

Thankfully, through my research I was prepared for these responses and did not allow them to diminish my desire or faith in my book. What did happen, though, was I stopped my daily writing and lost my momentum.

## *Quit waiting and start writing*

Once I stopped waiting to hear from the publishers, I started another waiting game. Waiting for the dishes to be done, the laundry caught up, and the social obligations to stop. Waiting for the perfect day, the perfect time, the perfect mood. Waiting for the impossible.

Then, finally, my waiting came to a grand finale when a dear friend and fellow writer sent me Brenda Ueland's book, *If You Want to Write.* (First copyrighted 1938!) Within the first few pages, my perception of writing as merely a sideline or hobby began to change.

I no longer had a choice. Writing simply had to become a top priority. That is, *if* I truly wanted my life to make a difference. Ueland said it perfectly:

> "We have come to think that duty should come first. I disagree. Duty should be a by-product. *Writing*, the creative effort, the use of the imagination, should come first — at least for some part of every day of your life. It is a wonderful blessing if you will use it. You will become happier, more enlightened, alive, impassioned, lighthearted and generous to everybody else. Even your health will improve. Colds will disappear and all the other ailments of discouragement and boredom."

*Voila!* That summed it up for me. The majority of us take our duties and obligations and place them at the center of our lives and give what little time we have left to recreation and resting. "Yes," you say, and I agree, these are crucial elements — working, nurturing our families, homework, sports and even leisure tme. But, without our creative dimension being discovered, developed, and then expressed, the rest adds up to a possibly decent and happy life, but a life where our unique talent is wasted, never expressed, never shared with the world.

In Agnes de Mille's memoir, *Dance to the Piper,* she quotes from her teacher, Martha Graham:

> "There is a vitality, a life force, a quickening that is translated through you into action, and because there is only one of you in all time, the expression is unique. And if you block it, it will never exist through any other medium...and be lost. The world will not have it.
>
> It is not your business to determine how good it is or how valuable it is; or how it compares with other expressions. It is your business to keep it yours clearly and directly. To keep the channel open.
>
> You do not even have to believe in yourself or your work. You have to keep open and aware directly to the urges that motivate YOU. Keep the channel open.... No artist is pleased.... There is no satisfaction whatever at any time. There is only a queer, divine dissatisfaction; a blessed unrest that keeps us marching and makes us more alive."

This quote liberated me from worrying about the value of my work and made me more determined to not block, "to not lose for all time," my ability or desire to express. It assured me that tuning-in to our unique talent will bring more vitality and meaning to our lives and thus to the lives of others. Whether you or I have great talent is not the issue. It is the contagiousness of our zest that counts.

This revelation that all people have a certain talent and a unique creative side has aided me greatly in facing the next half of my life. I am counting on it to keep me growing and centered.

I encourage all of you who take the time to read my words to stop running around doing this and that, as I have been doing for most of my life, and start doing or finding what it is that you and you alone have to offer this world. Do not worry how superb or pitiful others may find your creative effort — just express it as if your life depends on it.

Ueland claims in her book that Van Gogh's letter to his brother changed her life. He said (as quoted in her book):

> "In a few years I must finish a certain work. I need not hurry myself; there is no good in that-but I must work on in full calmness and serenity, as regularly and focused as possible, as briefly and concisely as possible. The world only concerns me in so far as I feel a certain debt and duty towards it and out of gratitude want to leave some souvenir in the shape of drawings or pictures — not made to please a certain tendency in art, but to express sincere human feeling."

Yes, you say, but this is Van Gogh. Even so, it is interesting that he wrote this letter when he was in his early twenties with no thought at that time of being an artist. He was studying to be a clergyman. And even after he began to paint, Van Gogh lived a life of poverty and starvation, depth and gratitude. He never knew his paintings would be worth millions of dollars one day. His paintings have been much more than the delightful souvenir he desired and he has led others to a deep understanding of art. As Euland says:

> "The moment I read Van Gogh's letter I knew what art was, and the creative impulse. It is a feeling of love and enthusiasm for something, and in a direct, simple, passionate and true way, you try to show this beauty in things to others, by drawing it."

Van Gogh's words changed Brenda Ueland's life. Her words changed my life. The closing of her book brings it all together for me:

> "And why should you do all these things? Why should we all use our creative power and write or paint or play music, or whatever it tells us to do? Because there is nothing that makes people so generous, joyful, lively, bold and compassionate, so indifferent to fighting and the accumulation of objects and money. Because, the best way to know truth or beauty is to try to express it. And, what is the purpose of existence here or yonder, but to discover truth and beauty and express it, i.e., share it with others?"

Funny, now when people ask "And what do you do?" I no longer have that pressure to impress others and myself with a great vocation. I simply say, "Oh, all sorts of things, but mostly I'm a mom, a wife and sometimes I write."

Seventeen

# Finding New Passions and Interests

*"You must do the thing you think you cannot do."*
Eleanor Roosevelt

As children, we were virtually *unplugged* from roles and responsibilities. Upon reaching adulthood, however, our sockets may have become so full that we needed an extension cord or two. Fortunately, midlife can provide us with the opportunity to clear out the extra clutter and chaos that stem from an over-loaded life and unfortunately, for many of us, a disease to please. Many of our previous roles are changing, even ending, and we can become wiser about what new roles we will take on.

If we are mothers, our children have grown up or at least have become more self-sufficient. Many of us have established careers or are thinking about new beginnings. Our social pressures may have diminished. We've learned to say no to unwanted obligations. And learning to detach from negative relationships provides us with additional time and energy as well.

Even though midlife naturally coincides with the automatic *unplugging* of some roles and expectations, there are still areas in our lives that will require us to manually and deliberately *unplug* – that is, if we truly want to emerge with a redefined sense of who we are and what we want to accomplish, and then have the time to go after it.

Sherry has probably taught me the most about the importance of pursuing new interests in our lives. Upon entering her forties, she found herself at a precarious point in her life. She realized two of her best friends had moved, her children didn't need her as much, and though her husband was basically wonderful (remember, the one she dumped my hubby for!), he was also a complete workaholic — to the point of using work as his recreation and leisure.

Sherry once asked him, "Rick, what do you enjoy most in life?"

Immediately he replied, "Weeding and cutting grass! "

O...kay. No wonder Sherry was beginning to sense a certain stagnation.

She wondered though, with a little guilt, what more could she ask for? She had a good marriage and three healthy children. Most probably the nurturing role she had been plugged in to for most of her life was simply getting old and void of newness. Her life was consumed with serving, not just her family, but her church, her clubs, her community, etc.

But instead of getting bogged down, Sherry began exploring areas that interested her. First, she asked for a mountain bike. Rick bought her one of the best on the market. She then proceeded to ride her mountain bike for miles and miles on the flat, dusty Delta turn rows. She was like a new person almost immediately.

I suppose her legs began to ache though, as the next thing we knew, she had bought a horse and instructed Rick to turn the greenhouse into a barn and to fence in the pecan orchard which of course, thrilled Rick to no end. He could get as dirty as he wanted and work for days and days on this project.

Anyway, to this day, Sherry amazes me as she occasionally fights the blues by finding new passions and interests to keep her awake and alive.

This is such an important ability for we women entering midlife. We must keep ourselves growing mentally, emotionally, spiritually and physically in order to keep the inevitable mundane from drowning us in its sheer predictability. And if the mundane has left us as we face the inevitable changes of life, whether it's grown up children, widowhood or divorce —then it's all the more crucial for us to begin anew by finding new areas of interest to pursue.

Again, my now deceased mother-in-law becomes a role model for me. Dane was just fifty-five when she became a widow. She lost her oldest son in an accident just a few years later.

Not long after these two tragedies ripped her world apart, she began taking painting and sculpturing classes. Upon looking back, Dane's children believe that her openness to express her creative side probably kept her sane during an incredibly sorrowful and challenging stage of her life. We are also blessed to this day to have beautiful souvenirs of her creative side that she left to us.

I thank God everyday that writing has come into my life. Waking up with a new purpose  has replenished within me a long lost sense of anticipation for what's to come. Even before I started this book I pursued new interests, and although they didn't pan out, so to speak — they kept me afloat.

For instance, I signed up for a two-month pottery course. I made several crooked bowls that I still treasure, but obviously it was not a strength of mine. I took a fly fishing course with my dear friend, Audrey,  that was wonderful. All of a sudden our hikes, which alone were a new passion for me, took on a new perspective. With our collapsible fly rods conveniently hooked onto the side of our backpacks, we could hike or ride horses up to a lake in the mountains and have the ability to fly fish for food or fun.

One of the greatest pleasures for me as I began to become *unplugged* was my newfound ability to take my horse for a ride instead of letting HIM take me for one. I had been scared to death of these huge, powerful animals ever since I had been thrown from one at Camp Greystone as a child. But, Carol, my friend in her sixties, showed me that if we encounter the very things we are afraid of then the fear diminishes.

I imagine this is what my heroine, Eleanor Roosevelt, meant in the quote at the head of this chapter. "You must do the thing you think you cannot do." I have this quote hanging next to my computer. It is carved in a piece of clay with a vine of leaves and flowers painted as a border around it.  Interesting — a famous woman who lived many years ago *said* it, a local woman *rewrote* it artistically and now I am encouraged to persevere daily as I *look* at it.

Again, this reminds me that anything we attempt to do which is from a creative impulse can not only enrich our own lives but bypass lifetimes and continue to be of influence to others.

*Eighteen*

# **Dangerous Distractions**

There is something lovely and natural about older women encouraging and teaching younger women.  My own life has been blessed many times by older friends willing to share their experiences and wisdom with me.

One of these friends, Alana, who is in her late fifties, has been a great inspiration to me — even though we've just been friends for a couple of years.  She is creative, spiritual and blessed with an abundance of positive energy.  She is the mother of two grown children and has been married to the neatest guy for over thirty years.

Today, I took her to lunch and we talked excitedly about the attributes of the *unplugged* woman. She is also a writer and we talked about our projects.

Then, over dessert, she suddenly decided to become very

*unplugged* herself and told me she has been having an affair for many, many years. "Years?" I asked, "Many, many years? You've been happily married for years!"

"Oh, no", I thought. My *unplugged* role model married all these years, is unfaithful to her husband, whom I know she loves deeply. So much for being unplugged. I felt electrocuted to the bone.

I asked, "How could you?" And then, "How did you?"

The logistics were not all that interesting, as her encounters with her lover were few and far between. But the utter pain and intense pleasure were another story. Contradictions again.

This is not good for me to hear at this time in my life. Yes, I'm finally getting it all together. But why do I also feel vulnerable? Is this *unplugging* I've been preaching dangerous? Will I *unplug* from my standards, morals and vows as well?

I was scared. I thought I was getting stronger. Strong enough to remain on my feet no matter how hard the wind blows. Yet, now I see that I will always have to bend with the breezes in life, and perhaps even get blown off my feet every now and then. I may fall to the ground and simply get the wind knocked out of me. Or maybe get caught up in a twister that keeps me frantically flying in a whirlwind of pleasure, panic and pain.

So, this is my question. If I'm still susceptible to losing my way, then what is the difference between the supposedly new and stronger me and the plugged-in weakling of yesterday?

I know there is something very important here for me to recognize. I think, I ponder...and then I see. I'm not necessarily more moral or better in my *unplugged* glory. I'm just more resilient, and a lot less judgmental.

My friend has been married for over three decades and I do believe her when she claims she loves her husband deeply. Nevertheless, she cares for another man as well. She may only see her other lover every now & then, but she admits her everyday life is immensely distracted by just the thought of him.

Alana is aware that it's a no-win situation. To her, it is something that went too far — one little itty-bitty step at a time — a long, long time ago.

I simply listened, and part of me understood, accepted and even appreciated the humanity of it all. I wondered how many of us are in the same situation — married to a person we love; yet simultaneously having another meaningful or not so meaningful relationship on the side. Or maybe some of us are haunted by memories of a past love affair. Or perhaps a fantasy that we must keep buried within us. Our spouses may have similar distractions.

Thankfully, one shining truth of great value came to me during my visit with Alana. Even in her vulnerability, her wisdom shined through as she taught me the value of continuity.

This is a concept I had never really considered until Alana

pointed it out to me. As she considered the possible consequences of her infidelity, she expressed that one of the most
tragic outcomes would be losing the continuity of her family.

Alana and her husband, Bob, have been building a life
together for over thirty years. She knows and loves his parents
and siblings. He knows and respects her parents and family. But
most importantly, they have raised two children together.

Alana said to me, "I imagine when our son decides to
marry. Will I walk down the aisle and sit alone or with my new
mate? Will Bob sit behind me or down the aisle from me — or
possibly with his new mate? Our son is getting married, and we
cannot even hold hands and share in the joy of it together."

Next, Alana had me imagining that her daughter had just
given birth to her first baby. If Alana and her husband are still
together, they will race to the hospital and simply walk in and
glow as they pass their first grandchild back and forth between
them.

But, what if Alana had chosen to leave him for her midlife
lover? At this point, all the natural and spontaneous reactions to
becoming grandparents must be constrained or at least organized. Due to the awkwardness, Alana may have to wait to see
her grandbaby until her ex and his new lady had their turn.

Sad, isn't it? To see a couple ditch their dreams that
they had built day by day for years, simply because one of them
was bored, neglected, or whatever, succumbed too quickly to

greener grass.

I know in one way, the beginning of my relationship with Hank was quite similar. Compared to my hectic life with Ron, his grass did appear greener! But, I see now how little continuity Ron and I had to fall back on. Hank and I treasure the years we have invested in our marriage and I believe if other couples would do the same, the susceptibility to stray would diminish greatly.

Someone once told me that a marriage is like a bank account. If you keep making withdrawals (insults, neglect, etc.) and not enough deposits (compliments, flowers, love, etc.), then it won't be long before the account is in the red...before there's nothing left. But if the deposits outweigh the withdrawals, then the marriage will have a strong foundation on which to stand — ever increasing. I wonder how much the concept of continuity is cherished.

*Nineteen*

# ***Inevitable Farewells***

*"She taught me by her actions, that one truly can make a difference in this world by doing simple things in consistent ways."*

Sallie Burdine

My mother-in-law was dying. She had been a huge part of my life for close to twenty years. Her name was Baby Jane. A classic Southern nick name that evolved from Narcissa Jane Rule. She was also known as "Dane" by her grandchildren, daughters-in-law and various others.

At eighty-seven years old, Dane had been blessed with excellent health until about a month before she died, when she became short of breath and we received the grim news that massive congestive heart failure was awaiting her in the near future.

"How can this be?" we silently screamed in desperation.

Dane was still gardening, entertaining and living her life to the fullest. In her spare time she worked crossword puzzles, which she claimed kept her mind alert. We, her children, grand-children and loved ones, wondered how we would ever go on without her.

Who would keep us all together? Who would feed the wild birds and ducks that had come to depend on her? Who would protect her beloved daylilies, irises and other perennials?

Dane's entire life had revolved around us — our comings and goings, our safety, our welfare. Every day for forty-some-thing years, she wrote in her journal the details of our lives, the blooming of her flowers and the status of the weather.

Our inward screaming soon stopped, and we began to prepare for her death. We started by celebrating her life and all that it stood for. Then we found gratitude that her final days would be painless and her passing would be quick.

About five weeks after the diagnosis, Dane was at home with her children and grandchildren hovering around her as she slowly faded away. She was very weak and close to the end of her physical life on earth. Our only comfort was that her pres-ence would live on in all of us and the legend of her beauty, strength and grace would be passed on for many generations.

From looking at photographs of Dane's younger years, it was easy to appreciate her attractiveness, but in her eighties, her beauty was unsurpassable. Her hair was reddish blonde, not white or gray, but naturally blonde and she wore it in a loose bun on top of her head. On the few occasions when we saw her with it down, we marveled at her shiny, thick, incredible hair that fell to her waist. Her large eyes were sapphire blue, and the lines on her face did little to detract from her loveliness. Her figure was slender, her style of dress was classic and she carried herself with cautious strength — until a few days before her death, when physical weakness sentenced her to bed. But even though Dane was not gracefully moving about anymore, her strength and love were still evident as she prepared to leave us.

We all took turns sitting next to her or laying with her as we held her hand and told her how much we loved her. We assured her that we would take care of each other and would feed the birds and keep her daylilies blooming forever. And in the quiet moments, I reflected on all the many lessons her exceptional life taught me.

As a woman who had endured incredible tragedy throughout her life, Dane continued to live each day with optimism and gratitude. In 1961, Dane's husband drowned while securing his boat during a storm. She was left with five small children, ages ten to eighteen, to raise on her own. Her oldest son was killed nine years later in a motorcycle accident. Within the next few years, she lost two sisters and two brothers, all resulting from sudden, tragic accidents. The list goes on and on.

The point is that, in spite of all the pain, Dane continued to appreciate the beauty and blessings of everyday life. She taught my children and me to be aware of and grateful for flying hawks, rain, rainbows and even blooming weeds. She inspired me to search for the art of living in the present.

As you know, I had struggled most of my pre-menopausal life to find a purpose or a mission in life. Dane taught me by her actions that one truly can make a difference in this world by doing simple things in consistent ways. Whether it is the hundreds of birds she fed over the years, or the endless planting of trees and flowers, Dane succeeded in nurturing the environment. The important thing is that she did it with the right motives and without any great sense of universal mission.

Dane also nurtured the human world with her daily invitations to the widowed, the lonely and the unwanted to come share a "toddy" with her. (She drank two scotch and milks daily for some fifty years). The invitations would continue until a guest would monopolize the conversation or talk while someone else was talking. If the guest was young, female and guilty of interrupting a gentleman, Dane would quietly take her into the kitchen and gently reprimand her. If the guest was older and should have known better, they would not be invited back.

Nevertheless, in spite of Dane's dominating spirit, I learned by watching her reach out to people that we really do reap what we sow. Dane's life was filled with people who loved and admired her in untold ways.

I am enormously thankful that my mother-in-law was in good health during my bout with instant menopause. Dane nursed me back to health after my hysterectomy. There she was, in her early eighties, helping with the children, the cooking and the cleaning.

I remember one evening in particular when the children were asleep and we decided to have a nightcap. Dane suggested I try a scotch and milk — to ease my pain and discomfort. I settled for a bourbon and milk, which was really quite soothing and then we began to indulge in our other nightcap...a game or two of Scrabble.

Dane had decided, in her later years, to stop keeping score and this put a damper on our Scrabble tournaments. Actually, it irritated the hell out of me...at least, the competitive me.

I once asked her, "Why, Dane? The game is much more satisfying if you know your score."

She quickly responded, "But why keep score? It doesn't matter who wins. It just matters that we play."

In looking back, I don't know why it bothered me; she was a pro and would have beaten the socks off of me anyway.

On that particular night, though, as we usually did, our conversations would drift and distract us as we tried to drum up miraculous words that would fill in the blanks on our Scrabble board.

I asked her if she had struggled mentally and/or physically during her change of life.

She said, "I don't really remember, but I know it's always best to just take two aspirin and think about someone other than yourself."

It has been about four years now since Dane died — on Mother's Day weekend.  A hospice team taught us how to let her go with peace and dignity.  It may sound strange, but she seems more alive and with us now than ever before.

The post-menopausal me continues to reflect, except with more clarity, on the many lessons my beloved mother-in-law taught me.  I wish I had learned them earlier, but I'm thankful I can grasp them now.

I realize that there are many parents who are not held in such high esteem in their older years or upon their death.  Many are also not blessed with such a painless and quick death as Dane's.

My grandmother, who was in her nineties, lived her final years in a nursing home.  She was scared, confused and tired of living for most of those years.  My mother and aunt lovingly, yet exhaustingly, took care of her for two decades.

My mother has battled breast cancer for almost fourteen years.  My father passed away rather suddenly due to heart problems.

Many of my close friends have lost parents in the last

year. This should not be surprising, for midlife is the time for the previous generation to become elderly. But, somehow I didn't realize so many of us would soon be grieving the loss of our parents, too. I was so caught up in other midlife issues that I was shocked at the enormity of this fact of life. Now I know that the increased probability of our parent's decline and potential deaths cannot be discounted.

For those of us with parents still living, we must prepare ourselves for the potential burden of having to take care of them. It's as if we will begin to parent our parents and this can cause frustration and resentment for all involved — our parents, ourselves, and our siblings, who may not be able or willing to share in the care-giving role.

In Paula Payne Hardin's insightful book, *What Are You Doing with the Rest of Your Life,* she stresses the importance of being prepared for this challenge that may soon confront us.

> "As parents come to the time of life when they need our help, we can expect to go through a transition ourselves. The relationship between adult children and their frail, elderly parents can be stressful, a tangle of anguish, frustration, devotion, guilt, and love.
>
> By engaging in preparation strategies such as reading books and talking with others before the crisis of aging, ill, or dying parents confronts us, we can begin to sort out our feelings and priorities while there is space and time to think clearly. We can educate ourselves about the options that are suitable for our circumstance."

She goes on to say:

"How our parents live their last years can be a profound experience for us, a time of reconciliation, perhaps, a time of increased intimacy. At the very least, it will be a learning experience from which we can benefit."

Twenty

# The Value of Solitude

*Loneliness is inner emptiness.*
*Solitude is inner fulfillment.*

> — Richard J. Foster
> *Celebration of Discipline*

Solitude?  How elusive this concept, even the very word, seems to me — aloneness. Time for just me.  To write, to walk, to read, or most of all to do nothing.  Mission impossible, I do be-lieve.  Yes, there are those occasional few hours or minutes during the day when something similar to solitude happens.  I have time to myself — but the cloud of time passing becomes my annoying companion.  You know, that awareness of things to come three hours before the kids are out of school, an appointment or whatever.  Then two hours, and then one hour...the clock is ticking faster.  I need to change clothes and put on some makeup if I'm going out. Or I need to get dinner started, or fold the clothes and on and on. Like I said, similar to solitude — but it just doesn't hit the mark.

Before my mother-in-law passed away, she told me to savor the noise and commotion because one day it would be gone, replaced by only quiet and fear of what I will do alone again each night. We always joked about changing places. She would come to visit and tend to the needs and wants of five people, the endless housework, and the telephone. I would go to her house and play solitaire, do crosswords and wish the phone would ring.

Funny, she always had her phone clipped to her clothes, just in case one of her children or grandchildren or lonely widow friends would call. I, on the other hand, turn off the ringer and listen to my messages maybe once or twice a day. In fact, I HATE the telephone these days. Loved ones and strangers with reasonably good intentions call and interrupt our life regularly. Not that I don't do the same to others.

My teenage niece, who has been living with us for many years, and my preteen son, cannot stay off the phone, and my husband is not much better. He enjoys surprise calls and loves to call others with the most trivial tidbits to share.

Maybe this annoyance is just a phase for me. Or maybe I am becoming permanently reclusive? Who knows? Who cares? I just wish the phone would become as *unplugged* as me.

I crave the quietness right now. Where does it fit in?

Prayer and meditation? No music? No writing? Even though my outer voice is silent, my inner voice is yakking endlessly. I suppose, as with everything, balance is the key...walking in nature with a silent mind, meditating as I allow my thoughts to float by like clouds in the sky. Then, when I indulge in creativity, my spirit may be cleansed of the unnecessary clutter and real truth can be found.

I begin to obsess on having days and days of solitude. Then I realize I am focusing on the lack of it and this will not work. So I visualize what I *want* instead of what I don't *have*. I know my "deliberate creation" will work. "As a man thinketh, so is he." The universe will respond to my thoughts.

A friend taught me this concept and it works just about every time. While I wait for the manifestation of my thoughts, I now receive peace instead of frustration. I now make the mental decision to trust and begin visualizing the possible outcomes. Maybe I'll escape to a retreat somewhere. But how will I pack my computer? Maybe the funds for a laptop will appear! Or maybe Hank and the kids will go away on a vacation...and simply leave me at home, all by myself.

I'll turn off the phone and maybe tell everyone I've gone off with my family so no one will drop in...except possibly burglars. No worries, though, I live in the mountains in a practically crime free area with four vicious canine "actors". Also, my husband's assorted hunting and trapshooting artillery should keep me safe. And if it snows, my seclusion will be guaranteed unless very fit cross-country skiers or snowshoers decide to venture up our mile long, uphill driveway.

But then, the guilt creeps in over leaving my family or not going with them on some special vacation where irreplaceable special memories will be made. And what would our friends think?

Oh, I forgot — I don't care anymore. I am *unplugged* from criticism. Now my thought processes are working right. My new way of living takes practice. I see improvement, though. It's as if there is another "I" living inside of me that is gently erasing my plugged-in blackboard of yesterday.

Spring break is coming up in about three weeks. Hank and I have planned a ten-day journey with our kids to visit dear friends in Houston, and then on to San Antonio. I've always wanted to go to the Riverwalk and the Alamo, plus Leukenback and Greune Hall, to see Jerry Jeff Walker. Then there's watching my kid's faces at Six Flags. Oh, dear. It will be interesting to see if I decide to go. Hank has already said, "Stay, write, and have your solitude."

Hank and the boys leave for the spring break trip. My daughter and niece stay with me. I have more solitude than usual, but the comings and goings of the people remaining put me on a schedule. The roles of chauffeur, cook, housekeeper, laundress and nurturer continue to be mine. I'm still visualizing the real thing.

Two months later, the kids finish school and start their summer break. They board our old motor home and leave with their wonderful dad to go to Mosquito-ville, Mississippi for two weeks! My niece has gone to spend the summer with her mother in Florida. I am the only human being on two hundred and fifty acres. I'm surrounded by dogs, cats, parakeets, horses, a goat, a burro and wildlife galore. They don't talk. Most of them just graze, and the others only need to be fed once a day.

Today begins my experiment with solitude. A long dose of aloneness for the first time in my life. My respite comes on the cusp of many years of increasing non-aloneness.

Last night, however, my elation eluded me totally. After my seven-year-old daughter fell asleep in my arms, I cried like a baby. She and I had talked softly as we cuddled before she drifted off to sleep.

I asked her if she knew why Mama wasn't going with them this time.

She said, "So you can have some peace...and so you can work on your book."

And then she said exactly what I had feared, "I hate your book, mama. It takes you away from me."

There it was — like a knife in my heart. I tried to explain to her why mama needs something more than just caring for her. I reminded her of how good she feels when she creates a picture or sets up her toy horses just right in their red barn. I told her that when she grows up, she would need to be creative and feel that same sense of accomplishment. She listened so sweetly and then just held me tighter. Soon she fell asleep as I fell apart.

I questioned my decision to stay while they all left. But, again, the words written by another put me back on track. I crept downstairs with my red, swollen eyes and began to read from a book that my friend, Julie, had just sent to me. Just as Brenda Ueland's words saved my motivation to keep writing, this author saved my gift of solitude from being ruined by guilt and regret.

Anne Morrow Lindbergh, in her book, *Gift from the Sea*, spoke to me directly. She said:

> "It is a difficult lesson to learn today — to leave one's friends and family and deliberately practice the art of solitude for an hour or a day or a week. For me, the break is the most difficult. Parting is inevitably painful, even for a short time. It is like an amputation, I feel. A limb is being torn off, without which I shall be unable to function.
>
> And yet, once it is done, I find there is a quality to being alone that is incredibly precious. Life rushes back into the void, richer, more vivid, and fuller than before. It is as if in parting one did actually lose an arm. And then, like the starfish, one grows it anew; one is whole again, complete and round — more whole, even, than before, when the other people had pieces of one."

I was comforted immediately. The parting *is* the worst part. Once they left and more tears were shed, I walked stoically into the house, looked around at its emptiness and shouted, "YES!" My amputated loving limb was cruising down the driveway as my new limb was growing back at full speed.

I have been alone for several days now and I am frightened. Not of being alone, mind you, but by how much I love being alone. It's as if a gift surpassed by none other has been bestowed upon me.

## *Silence*

The first few days I had to have music playing constantly. I have now learned that without silence there is no solitude. I have opened the windows in my writing room, and in my endeavor to find silence I am hearing more. In fact, all of my senses seem to have come alive. The wind blowing and the birds singing soothe my previously frazzled spirit.

I am not speaking now, except to the animals a little. Weaning myself from the telephone, the very thing I most resent has been the hardest. Of course, I have to touch base with Hank and the kids, but not talking to my soul sisters has been especially difficult. I didn't realize how addicted I am to frantically spewing out words and hearing them as well. I hope that, when my vacation from reality is over, I will be more conscious of how much I talk.

In *Celebration of Discipline*, Richard J. Foster writes:

*"The tongue is our most powerful weapon of manipulation. A frantic stream of words flows from us because we are in a constant process of adjusting our public image. We fear so deeply what we think other people see in us, so we talk in order to straighten out their understanding."*

Aha! Do I ever relate to that!

## Steps Into Everyday Solitude

My family will be returning soon and I am determined to become more disciplined in maintaining some of this precious solitude.

I also plan to take longer than mere moments for myself. Maybe a few hours every week, a day every month, I hope, at least one full week each year. I know this may be tough for some people economically, but I am convinced where there is a will, there is a way.

One of the best substitutes I have found for immediate solitude is a long soak in a bath tub. I tell everyone in the house that I'm going to take a bath and basically, to leave me alone. They know this means "Do Not Disturb."

I put on some soft instrumental music, light some candles, and emerge thirty minutes to an hour later as a new woman. A little sleepy and over-protective of my renewal but relaxed and refreshed, nevertheless.

## The fruit of solitude

My seemingly selfish pursuit of solitude has already contrasted itself in an unselfish desire to truly "be" with the people
in my life. I am rested now, stronger and more centered. I am
ready to be a mom, a wife, and a friend...again. My sensitivity
and compassion for others is greater as well.

I have decided to be two, maybe three people in this
second half of my life. What's wrong with multiple personalities,
anyway? I want to be zestful, vibrant, enthusiastic, and yes, I
admit—beautiful and a little glamorous, as well. The other me
will be a listener, a lover of all people-void of prejudice, judgment and vanity — okay, maybe not vanity. But, I *will* shed my
makeup every now and then and venture into the wilderness to
soak up the nourishment of nature. My objective will be to find
peace sans guilt with all of these personas—to be *unplugged from*
any certain roles yet still adhere to my responsibilities.

*Twenty-one*

## *Alone Together —*
## *Interruption or Enhancement?*

*"It is easy in the world to live after the world's opinion; it is easy in solitude to live after our own, but the great man is he who in the midst of the crowd keeps with perfect sweetness the independence of solitude."*

— Ralph Waldo Emerson
*"Self-Reliance"*

I have four days left to myself. Mary Ellen calls to inform me she is flying in to Denver to get away from it all as her divorce drags on. She offers to rent a car and do her own exploring without bothering my solitude. I decide it is time to leave my beloved yet, empty nest and take a break from writing. I also want to be with my friend. We have a way of being "alone together" which is another kind of solitude.

So I pack my bags and Audrey's boxer, Maya, who I am

dog-sitting for six weeks while Audrey is showing off her new baby to her family in Europe. I have watched Maya grow from a puppy who was unbearable to ride in a car with — barking constantly at everything — to a mature three year old who now merely *observes* as she cruises. Of course, Maya has never known she is canine, at least, until Audrey gave birth to a human three months ago. Now she is finding her true identity as she relates to my dogs and other animals at Camp *Burdine*.

Even so, Maya remains too special to stay behind in the pen with my other dogs. She also has epilepsy and needs human attention in the midst of her occasional seizures. So I pack her fleece bed, special bowls, food, toys, etc. and off we go to pick up Mary Ellen at the airport. The three of us then proceed to cruise in the mountain towns west of Denver.

After a couple of days, we decide to head home by taking the back roads and being spontaneous to any detours along the way. One of our detours is to drive through the gambling town of Cripple Creek where we stop to walk and water Maya. We pay $5.00 in order to park, which was refundable if we went into one of the Saloon-looking casinos — which we did. After receiving our $5.00 back in quarters we decided to throw it back into a slot machine named "Dazzling Double Sapphires" which the two Virgos in us could not resist. We hit a couple of small jack pots which kept us playing for an hour or so and then finally lost everything, including an extra twenty or thirty dollars.

As we left, a little old lady at the door recommended that we drive through Phantom Canyon instead of taking the regular route home. She said it was the same distance, just more interesting. So, of course, without any hesitation we chose to be a little bit contrary to the ordinary.

Little did I know we were about to enter the Twilight Zone for two hours, when the other way would have taken thirty minutes. We turned right instead of the usual left and began descending down red, clay, gravel roads into the most incredible canyons and crevices. The road began narrowing and winding until we realized this was not a road for wimps. We tried with difficulty and amusement to imagine the little old lady at the Casino maneuvering her car down this pass she had recommended to us.

Not that it wasn't beautiful... It was late afternoon and the low sun made everything look a deep, translucent, rusty red color—except for the trees and sky. Giant boulders and rocks protruded all around us. We stopped to use Mother Nature's bathroom and as we squatted and dripped dry we looked anxiously around us for mountain lions, rattlesnakes and Grizzly bears.

We were in awe, even Maya seemed spell struck—at least, until the empty gas alarm went off and we realized we had not looked at the gas gauge for two days. Damn, we were on empty. I mean, not even in the red, we were on E! The little gas pump icon on my dashboard was buzzing and there we were...in the middle of nowhere.

We estimated we were half way through Phantom Canyon and only had about twenty miles to go until the next town, so we decided to just keep going instead of turning back. It also helped that we were heading downhill and could coast most of the way.

Another problem arose when the sky began to change with urgency, as it so often does in the Rockies. Our bright blue ceiling began to pale as light gray, then dark charcoal gray clouds began to enclose us in our red canyon. The temperature dropped to forty degrees. The wind picked up and we knew a fierce hailstorm could hit at any minute.

Mary Ellen was at the wheel and continued to maneuver the twists and turns with skill as we coasted our way down. We were a little panicky, though, while keeping up our speed, which meant careening around some curves in order to avoid braking too much and ending up at a complete stop.

We began to take stock of our provisions as we realized there was a good possibility we may be spending the night in Phantom Canyon. Walking the extra ten to fifteen miles to civilization was no longer an option as nighttime and a hailstorm closed in.

It became immediately apparent that we basically had no provisions to speak of. Somehow these two usually smart women had not only overlooked the need to keep the gas tank filled but we neglected to bring a cell phone, foul weather gear, and even spare water and food. Maya had just finished the last of her water and had eaten her last meal early that morning.

Even so, we found comfort in discovering a warm unopened bottle of champagne from the day before. I searched through Mary Ellen's stuff as she continued to drive...I mean, coast and careen—only to find an airline size bag of peanuts and two old, crumbly Valium. We vowed to one another that when we really got cold, scared and hungry we would split the Valium and champagne with Maya.

After five or ten minutes more of coasting and trying to keep our wits about us, we turned a curve and saw an old, dilapidated mirage-looking gas station and house. "Yes!" We shouted. If nothing more, we found shelter and we hoped, gas, food and a phone, as well. As we pulled into the driveway, a scraggly little man walked slowly out the door of the gas station.

Before we could say a word, he smiled at us with his ONE tooth and said, "Sorry, ladies, I'm slap out of gas." Mary Ellen then said, "We are, too."

I looked at her and almost said "No!" but held my tongue. Things were tense enough with Maya barking her head off at the man and looking like she was on the verge of having a seizure.

I asked him if he had any water and he pointed over to a faucet on the side of his house. We got Maya's water bottle out and some empty cups and walked with the man to the faucet. He turned on the water and out gushed red, I mean "RED" water.

Mary Ellen and I looked dishearteningly at one another.

The man said, "Don't worry, it may look funny, but it sho' makes you healthy."

We filled up Maya's bottle and to our surprise, our car started and even made it five more miles to a Texaco in Canon City.

Mary Ellen and I are still not sure if the man and the gas station were real or a mirage. We also wonder if maybe aliens had abducted us. Such a strange day....

The next morning, Maya and I drove Mary Ellen to the airport and returned home for two more days of "real" solitude. Being "alone together" with my soul sister was, as usual, something to remember.

## Twenty-two

# Loving Ourselves –
# A toast to you and me!

Well, here's to us, girls!  We are incredible women. Our minds, bodies and souls are absolutely beautiful and always have been. Let us accept and admire ourselves as little girls, teenagers, young women, and now as middle-aged women. Let us promise to love ourselves as old women, too.

We should be grateful that after all these years, many of us realize our true selves were stifled along the way.  Some of us even felt submerged into dark, deep wells...where the cork of our true nature — our SOULS — never seemed able to float to the surface and bob around freely.

What in the world was belittling enough to anchor down lighthearted buoys like us? Could it have been the rejection, the criticism, or the pressure to conform? Did our once zestful corks become more like sponges absorbing the negativity around us?

The heaviness of it all must have slowly, but surely, cast us downward into the murky depths of what were once the clear and pristine waters of our youth. Our true selves simply could not ascend until we quietly and prayerfully began to love and nurture ourselves. It was then that forgiveness and compassion became like a raft— holding us up as the tears of sorrow and loss seemed to flow endlessly at first. But soon, these tears were replaced with tears of relief and joy. The real woman inside all of us became *unplugged* from any falsehoods we might have had. We began to see glimpses of the little girls we used to be and still are.

Yes, we have all been very brave to begin truly loving ourselves. To even meet our own eyes in a mirror and *greet* them was a grand beginning. Now we are able to give ourselves as a gift to others— whole and unbroken.

We shall never forget this lesson:

>*"If we do not nurture ourselves first, then we will never nurture those around us."*

Scripture tells us to "love our neighbors as we love our-selves." So let us say, "I love you" to ourselves every day and feel the love for others within us grow. Scripture also says, "As a man thinketh, so is he." So let us think of ourselves as *wonder-ful*

and then sit back and watch ourselves become *full of wonder.*
Remember the words of Nelson Mandela:

> "And as we let our own light shine, we unconsciously give
> other people permission to do the same."

*So now you have it girls — unplug from the negatives
and unnecessities and may your own authentic light shine
evermore!*

# *Epilogue*

## by Hank Burdine

I have often been accused of going through a midlife crisis by abandoning my roots and leaving my beloved Mississippi Delta to take up residency elsewhere. Sallie says I did not leave the Delta—I simply brought it with me. This sense of belonging, while simultaneously being able to move and change, inspired me to write the epilogue for my wife's book, which essentially is a story about transformation.

I am a dyed-in-the-wool type of person. I don't like change. However, I have enough sense about me to know that change is inevitable. And the mark of a true man is how he adapts to that change, whatever it may be.

During my younger and single years, I was quite a carouser. However, I was always searching for that one particular and perfect woman that would fulfill my dreams. I was who I was, *by God,* and nobody was ever going to change that. I just needed the right partner to ride along with me. I did not want to marry just to be divorced several years later as so many of my friends had done. I wanted a guarantee that I would live happily ever after and that nothing would change, *period.* Of course, I soon found out that you get no guarantees in life and change is always just around the corner.

Any man worth his salt is going to have to realize that those women he holds most dear to him are going to change. This is a physiological given. Nothing stays the same. Her moods, her ambitions, her attractiveness, and her physical well being all will undergo dramatic alterations as she navigates the middle years of her life.

The best thing a man can do during this phase of life is to not only try to understand what is happening, but to be an integral part of this phase. Don't think, as I almost did, "Here we go again!"

When Sallie started to become noticeably concerned about various aspects of our marriage, it took a pretty strong awakening on my part to realize that maybe I needed to examine myself. If there was something I could do to make life more exciting or simply better, then any effort on my part would certainly be worth it.

A woman will change all during her years from puberty

through early adulthood and on to menopause. As I learned from Sallie, the *real* woman does not appear until most all of the facets of life are complete. She can then relate to true life experiences to help her make decisions that will guide her through the rest of her life.

Sallie has become a different person. She no longer listens and reacts to the whims and wishes of every friend. She no longer has to make up an excuse when she doesn't want to do something. She does what she wishes for the benefit and bet-terment of herself and her family. And people don't belittle her because of this change in her attitude—they admire her for her tenacity and level-headedness.

The changes Sallie has experienced since her "instant menopause" have enabled her to look at life with a different perspective. She now asks herself, "What do *I* think?" instead of "What would other people think?" She is her own woman and responds with an air of self-determination and background. The hill may appear too steep to climb, but with her experiences, she will try to be a better person whether she makes it to the top or not. She continues to grow and expand her horizons while beck-oning others to join the ride!

I could have stayed the same as I was and thought this was just another set of the "crazies," but I decided to see if I could also become a better person, or at least a little more enlightened during this phase of Sallie's life. What a blast! What a ride I am having!

The conversations are deeper, the hugs are longer, the vacations are more enjoyable, and the reason we do things are a little more off the wall. We know our profound love for each other has proven successful over the years and we want to nurture it. I hope and pray that it will only grow stronger and deeper.

I am afraid of what would have happened had I become narrow-minded and decided to not change along with Sallie. Thank God I got on board for the ride.

I am not saying that a man must now try to keep up with the woman in his life. However, he must realize that if she looks at this phase of her life as a learning opportunity, then he must also try and be an open-minded mate and go where two minds will lead. Sex will never be better, understandings of each other will be deeper and the union you both have formed will be stronger.

So, I would tell my men friends, "Try to understand your women, give them the freedom to think and be someone they have always felt they were, yet, were afraid somewhat to be. These girls are our backbones and if you want to have the time of your life, *UNPLUG* yourself, and be the free spirit you know you are, too! Go for it, and you will find a willingness and zest for life with your mate that you did not know was out there!"

And to my lady friends... Don't look back! Use this time of your life to be adventurous, smell the roses, nurture what is dear to you and know that you are a woman of the highest order, based on all that you have learned along the way. The symphony is now complete. It only needs fine-tuning and playing in harmony with all the other facets of your life. Don't get bogged down. Jump over the hurdles and keep on running — the race is now in the turn with a whole lot of living left. Make the best of it!